**Feminist Technosciences**

*Rebecca Herzig and Banu Subramaniam, Series Editors*

# Gender before Birth

SEX SELECTION in a
TRANSNATIONAL CONTEXT

**RAJANI BHATIA**

UNIVERSITY OF WASHINGTON PRESS
*Seattle*

*Gender before Birth* was made possible in part by a grant from the
Initiatives for Women Endowment Fund at the University at Albany.

University of Washington Press
www.washington.edu/uwpress

Library of Congress Cataloging-in-Publication Data
Names: Bhatia, Rajani, author.
Title: Gender before birth : sex selection in a transnational context / Rajani Bhatia.
Description: Seattle : University of Washington Press, [2018] | Series: Feminist
    technosciences | Includes bibliographical references and index. |
Identifiers: LCCN 2017048981 (print) | LCCN 2017053762 (ebook) |
    ISBN 9780295742946 (ebook) | ISBN 9780295999203 (hardcover : alk. paper) |
    ISBN 9780295999210 (pbk. : alk. paper)
Subjects: LCSH: Sex preselection—Social aspects. | Human reproductive
    technology—Social aspects. | Sex of children, Parental preferences for. |
    Feminism. | Science—Social aspects.
Classification:
    LCC QP279 (ebook) | LCC QP279 .B43 2018 (print) | DDC 174.2/8—dc23
LC record available at https://lccn.loc.gov/2017048981

Portions of this book were previously published in Rajani Bhatia, "Constructing
Gender from the Inside Out: Sex-Selection Practices in the United States," *Feminist
Studies* 36, no. 2 (2010), 260–291; Rajani Bhatia, "Cross-Border Sex Selection: Ethical
Challenges Posed by a Globalizing Practice," *IJFAB: International Journal of Feminist
Approaches to Bioethics* 7, no. 2 (2014), 185–218; and Rajani Bhatia, "A Reproductive
Justice Perspective of the Purvi Patel Case," *IJME: Indian Journal of Medical Ethics* 1,
no. 4 (2016), 249–253. Reprinted with permission from *Feminist Studies*, University
of Toronto Press (www.utpjournals.com), and IJME.

For Axel, Malvina, and Milan

# Contents

# Acknowledgments

I am indebted to my informants, who took the time out of their busy schedules to share their professional experiences. They patiently explained the technical aspects of their work in detail. I appreciate their time and their contributions to this study.

I also thank the editor in chief of the University of Washington Press, Larin McLaughlin, and the Feminist Technoscience series editors, Banu Subramaniam and Rebecca Herzig, for seeing the potential in this work and for their enduring and generous support of a first-time book author. I am grateful to the anonymous readers for their painstaking, constructive, and most of all positive (for which I am eternally grateful) reviews. I thank others at the University of Washington Press—Niccole Coggins, Beth Fuget, and Margaret Sullivan, among others—all of whom helped bring this book to completion. Sue Carter, the copy editor, made the writing so much clearer.

For their insights into and contributions to my research at the University of Maryland, I thank Bonnie Thornton Dill, Laura Mamo, Michelle Rowley, Carole McCann, and Linda Aldoory. I am grateful also to my colleagues at the University at Albany—Janell Hobson, Vivien Ng, Barbara Sutton, and Virginia Eubanks—for their collegiality and mentorship. For their smarts, inspiration, and camaraderie, I thank Bettina Judd, Mel Michelle Lewis, Ana Perez, Gwen D'Arcangelis, Lisa Campo-Engelstein, Anne Hendrixson, Betsy Hartmann, Marcy Darnovsky, Nalini Visvanathan, Manisha Gupte, Jade Sasser, and Ellen Foley. For hosting me during my research trip to Guadalajara, I thank my dear friend Jennifer Dorroh and her family.

Funding provided by the New York State/United University Professions Joint Labor-Management Committees through a Dr. Nuala McGann Drescher Affirmative Action/Diversity Leave Program afforded me the time during the fall of 2016 to complete data analysis and writing. Additionally, funding from the Research Foundation for the State University of New York supported research travel and expenses in later stages of this project. Initiatives for Women Endowment Fund at the University at Albany supported professional indexing. I extend further thanks to *Feminist Studies* for permission to reproduce some of my initial thoughts on this topic in the introduction, the *International Journal of Feminist Approaches to Bioethics* for parts of chapter 3 on cross-border sex selection, and the *Indian Journal of Medical Ethics* for my interpretation of the Purvi Patel case in chapter 4.

For nurturance, affection, and forever squelching all my doubts, I thank my partner, Axel Guerin. For making my home such a wonderful, grounding, and musical place I thank my children; and for their unconditional love, support, and wisdom throughout this project, I thank Wizie Bhatia Eads, Nam Bhatia, Nelida Deluchi, Rizie Kumar, and Naomi Hayman.

# Abbreviations

## Organizational Abbreviations

| | |
|---|---|
| ACOG | American College of Obstetricians and Gynecologists |
| ACRJ | Asian Communities for Reproductive Justice |
| ANSIRH | Advancing New Standards in Reproductive Health |
| ARS | Agricultural Research Service |
| ASRM | American Society for Reproductive Medicine |
| CDC | Centers for Disease Control and Prevention |
| CGS | Center for Genetics and Society |
| CHR | Center for Human Reproduction (New York) |
| CWPE | Committee on Women, Population, and the Environment |
| ESHRE | European Society of Human Reproduction and Embryology |
| FASDSP | Forum against Sex Determination and Sex Preselection |
| FDA | US Food and Drug Administration |
| FFWH | Forum for Women's Health |
| FIGO | International Federation of Gynecology and Obstetrics |
| FINRRAGE | Feminist International Network of Resistance to Reproductive and Genetic Engineering |
| GIVF | Genetics & IVF Institute (Fairfax, VA) |
| HFEA | Human Fertilisation and Embryology Authority |
| ICPD | International Conference on Population and Development (Cairo, Egypt, 1994) |
| NAACP | National Association for the Advancement of Colored People |
| NAPAWF | National Asian Pacific American Women's Forum |
| OHCHR | United Nations Human Rights Office of the High Commissioner |

| OTT | Office of Technology Transfer, Agriculture Research Service, USDA |
| SAALT | South Asian Americans Leading Together |
| UBINIG | Unnayan Bikalper Nitinirdharoni Gobeshona (Policy Research for Development Alternatives) |
| UN Women | United Nations Entity for Gender Equality and Empowerment of Women |
| UNFPA | United Nations Population Fund |
| UNICEF | United Nations Children's Fund |
| USDA | US Department of Agriculture |
| USPTO | US Patent and Trademark Office |
| WHO | World Health Organization |

## Technical Abbreviations

| AI | artificial insemination |
| ART | assisted reproductive technology |
| CGH | comparative genomic hybridization |
| FISH | fluorescence in situ hybridization |
| ICSI | intracytoplasmic sperm injection |
| IUI | intrauterine insemination |
| IVF | in vitro fertilization |
| NIPT | noninvasive prenatal blood tests |
| NRTs | new reproductive technologies |
| PCR | polymerase chain reaction |
| PGD | preimplantation genetic diagnosis |
| PGS | preimplantation genetic screening |
| PND | prenatal diagnostic technologies |

# Gender before Birth

# Introduction

## Lifestyle Sex Selection

IN THE EARLY TO MID-1990S, JUST AFTER THE END OF THE COLD War, an ambitious series of international conferences laid out forward-looking strategies for protecting the environment, promoting economic and social development, and safeguarding women's and human rights. Within this optimistic context, declarations from the International Conference on Population and Development (Cairo, 1994) and the World Conference on Women (Beijing, 1995) defined prenatal sex selection as an "act of violence against women," "a form of discrimination against the girl child," and "unethical" (UNFPA 1995, UN Women 1996). The documents called upon nation-states to prevent and eliminate prenatal sex selection. The language on sex selection arrived in the concluding documents of these international conferences for the first time and in strong connection to the culminating effort of global feminist activism to highlight and develop strategies to stop harm from abusive population policies. In the final decade of the twentieth century, UN structures with the fanfare of their themed conferences invited unprecedented levels of nongovernmental participation, giving feminists the opportunity to create coalitions across substantial geographic distances and an ability to impact international agendas. In the case of the 1994 International Conference on Population and Development (ICPD), held in Cairo, feminist coalitions aimed to replace narrowly defined fertility decline population policy with sexual and reproductive health and rights programs that explicitly condemn the use of coercion (Connelly 2008).

Ironically, at the very same moment in the western hemisphere, the institutional review board of the fertility clinic Genetics & IVF Institute (GIVF) in Fairfax, Virginia, approved the use of MicroSort, a preconception method of sex selection under trial for "family balancing." The company introduced the term *family balancing* to mean a practice by which married, heterosexual couples try to increase the probability of having an additional child of a sex less represented among their current children. GIVF opened the clinical trial of MicroSort to the nonmedical indication of "family balancing" to more fully realize the market potential of a new technology.

In other words, just as the international community came together to condemn sex selection, a fertility clinic in the United States created an ethical opening to the practice. The juxtaposition of these concurrent events signifies a major preoccupation of this book, which focuses on the co-constitution since the 1990s of a global form of stratified sex selection and new sex selection practices within "Fertility Inc." Feminist sociologist Laura Mamo uses this term to convey the competitive, for-profit, and relatively unregulated "big business" market of assisted reproductive technology (ART), especially as it manifests in the United States (Mamo 2010, 178). As an institutional complex, Fertility Inc. indicates larger economic privatization and globalization processes at work that have transformed biomedicine in a neoliberal era (Clarke et al. 2010, 53).

The United States plays a significant role in the science and practice of new forms of sex selection. In the mid to late 1990s, MicroSort, along with another new technology, preimplantation genetic diagnosis (PGD), began to be applied to sex selection in humans for purposes other than disease avoidance on US turf, where the practice is not illegal. MicroSort involves sorting sperm based on the chromosomes determinative of sex and using the sorted samples either with in vitro fertilization (IVF) or intrauterine insemination (IUI). MicroSort was part of a human clinical trial in the US from 1993 to 2012, at first only for medical indications but quickly expanding to "family balancing." In 2010 the US Food and Drug Administration (FDA) prohibited further nonmedical application of MicroSort in the trial, but the clinic corporation that sponsored the trial (GIVF) had by then already established laboratory sites abroad from which sorted sperm could enter international circuits, where off-label uses could continue unmonitored.

PGD is a broader diagnostic technology that can screen embryos for a number of chromosomal and genetic conditions, only a few of which are sex linked (such as Duchenne's muscular dystrophy and hemophilia). From the beginning of PGD's advance in human medicine in the 1980s in the UK, scientists, ethicists, and policy makers distinguished between medical and nonmedical applications of PGD, legitimizing only the former. In medical sex selection, PGD is used to prevent sex-linked diseases; in nonmedical sex selection, PGD involves testing embryos produced through IVF for the characteristic of sex and then preselecting embryos for implantation based on sex preference. Since both MicroSort and PGD are applied before pregnancy in conjunction with ART, they can circumvent the politically contentious abortion issue. The importance of this feature in the US context, where the legalization of abortion in 1973 elicited a strong backlash and the formation of an anti-abortion stronghold in US political and cultural life, cannot be overstated. To highlight this, I refer to this set of technologies as *sex selective ART*.

Sex selection expanded an already highly inaccessible, high-end, privatized market niche in ART to fertile consumers with an ability to pay out of pocket for its services. As quoted in *Fortune* magazine, an analyst at OrbiMed Advisors estimated a $200–$400 million per year market for MicroSort (Wadman 2001). However, the expense and rigorous processes involved—not to mention questions around legality and ethics—precluded mass dissemination and use. During the fifteen years—from 1995 to 2010—when MicroSort was available in the US for "family balancing," only 4,610 couples (92.2 percent of all users of the technique) enrolled for that indication (Karabinus et al. 2014, 6). Less is known about sex selective PGD. The Centers for Disease Control and Prevention (CDC) began collecting data on PGD in 2004, but that data does not break down into reasons for use. From 2005 to 2014, PGD use hovered between 4 and 6 percent of all IVF cycles (CDC 2016). However, for some clinics the proportion of IVF cycles employing PGD is far greater than these overall figures would suggest. Two US clinics in my study, for example, recorded rates of 86 and 62 percent in 2014 (CDC 2016, Stapleton 2015). Clearly, neither MicoSort nor PGD could revolutionize the field of reproductive medicine in the same way or to the same extent as the ultrasound scanner, yet, as I will show, their normalization provokes new meanings that fundamentally impact how we think about reproduction in the twenty-first century.

## The Normalization of Sex Selective ART

Mass print and television media in the United States heralded the emergence of these technologies as the answer to a long quest for scientifically proven methods for selecting the sex of a child. At the same time, prospective consumers of sex selection increasingly found each other on the internet, developing a collective identity based on their desire for a child of a particular sex. Patient/consumer activism via the internet provided sympathetic, self-help spaces that allowed individuals to express their intention to preselect offspring's sex or their disappointment at bearing or birthing a child of the "wrong sex." Taken together, these developments signaled a new era in which the desire to choose having a male or female baby became "biomedicalized," or increasingly normalized as an *indication* to intervene medically for sex selection.

I was an interested observer of these developments. In the mid-1990s activists from the Forum for Women's Health (FFWH) in Mumbai, India, first brought the issue of sex selection to my attention. Their history of engagement in a movement against sex selection in India strongly affected my own feminist framing of the issue. Founding members of FFWH had in 1985 become alarmed by increasing evidence of what they defined as a "misuse" of prenatal diagnostic technologies such as amniocentesis or ultrasound scanning for sex selection. Son preference motivated the alarming growth in the practice of sex selective abortion of female fetuses. Women's movements in India quickly took up the issue because they viewed sex selection as a form of violence against women and girls, threatening their very survival. Together with other activists from people's science, health, human rights, and legal action organizations and movements, they formed the Forum against Sex Determination and Sex Preselection (FASDSP). Significantly, FASDSP formulated its primary objective not in terms of passing judgment on the technologies themselves but in terms of a broader opposition to all forms of discrimination against girls and women (Contractor et al. 2003, 9).

I first encountered the issue of sex selection in the US in the early fall of 2001, when the *New York Times* reported (erroneously, as it turns out) that the Ethics Committee of the American Society for Reproductive Medicine (ASRM) had approved the use of PGD for nonmedical sex selection (Kolata 2001). Just a month prior, the same newspaper reported the targeting of sex selection advertisements to South Asian communities in newspapers such as the North American editions of *India Abroad* and *Indian Express* (Sachs 2001). The juxtaposition of these two articles moved me into an advocacy mode, jumpstarted through a protest letter campaign directed to members of the ASRM Ethics Committee. My activist involvement in a campaign to raise concerns about the practice of sex selection lasted about four years, but my engagement with the issue did not end there.

When I campaigned on sex selection in the early 2000s, we interpreted the issue within a reproductive justice frame because of its indelible ties to quintessential examples of reproductive oppression named by scholars and activists at that time, such as sterilization abuse, coercive contraception, and unjust population control policies. A feminist critique of population control led to a conceptualization of reproductive justice and became one of its grounding stakes. The critique raised the specter of misuse of birth control technologies to limit rather than expand the reproductive freedoms of some groups of women (Hartmann 1995, Roberts 1997). Thus, an awareness of the global injustices of population control anchored our interpretation of sex selection within a framework of reproductive justice and contributed to our growing outrage at a market that could profit while exacerbating gender-based violence among particular subgroups of the national population. The idea that some women might feel compelled to "choose" a sex selective abortion due to combined pressures to reduce family size and bear sons challenged the idea of choice at the heart of reproductive rights struggles in the US. We knew better than to expect that mainstream reproductive rights organizations would willingly take up, let alone center, sex selection as an issue of concern.

Later, as a scholar, I continued to follow the issue closely for another eleven years. Long after my activist involvement receded, the campaign that I had helped start continued via different organizations and new actors. Over time its goals shifted in response to changing political realities, most pressingly the emergence of sex selective abortion bans proposed by anti-abortion groups in the US beginning in 2008. While on a practical level, FASDSP in India back in the 1980s looked for ways to stem the practice without curbing the legal right to abortion, in the United States even condemning the practice became fraught with the potential of playing into an anti-abortion agenda that reinforced harmful stereotypes about Asians.

This book stems from insights I have gathered over travels across time and space—over fifteen years both as an activist within international women's health movements and transnational feminist networks and as an interdisciplinary scholar in women's, gender, and sexuality studies.

In addition to a multimethod approach to fieldwork, I draw on experience developed through feminist practice in India, Germany, and the US, transnational feminist theory, and feminist thought on science and technology to develop a unique analysis that brings together empirically observed practices of reproduction alongside interpretation of their representation.

The book presents new empirical material gained during my lengthy engagement with the issue, which steered me into many sites as both participant and nonparticipant observer, including US ART clinics that have heavily marketed sex selection, the US Department of Agriculture, and the American Society for Reproductive Medicine's annual conference. The research follows MicroSort and PGD as they form a set of related practices in their material, discursive, and institutional travels both within and across national borders. The study combines inquiry into multiple social worlds, on- and off-line sites, and written and visual texts, all as they relate to the institutional center of practice in the ART clinic.[1]

Collected mainly from the 2010 to 2011, and then during the summer of 2015, data also stem from interviews I conducted with clinic directors, nurses, embryologists, and lab technicians primarily at two US ART clinics, as well as in US laboratory and clinical satellite locations in Mexico. I also interviewed self-help book and website authors, nongovernmental organization (NGO) representatives advocating on the issue of sex selection, the scientific director of the MicroSort investigative trial in the United States, and a fertility clinic CEO in Nigeria. Although two self-help authors offered some insights on their successful experiences using sex selective ART (one used MicroSort to have a girl and the other PGD to have a boy), I did not solicit their input to the study as users of the technologies, but as authors of books or websites. Thus, I do not represent or interrogate the subjective experience of sex selective ART users. Rather, I query the organization and institutional mechanisms that brought forth the practice from the perspective mainly of providers.

Drawing on transnational feminist theory and the methodologies of feminist scholars, who combine grounded analyses of material, discursive, and institutional formations, I trace how these three simultaneously occurring processes configured the anticipation of lifestyle sex selection, its incorporation into Fertility Inc., its extension through global networks, and finally its contestation among various interested groups. I interrogate the truth and knowledge claims about sex selective ART as they are defined in relation to abortion practices.

## The Politics of Naming: "Sex," "Selection," and "Lifestyle"

In the early 2000s, as I grappled with the way the issue unfolded in the US, I found it baffling to make sense of information that campaign members circulated—the news media articles, the advertisements, and the blogs. I was unsettled by the rhetoric of freedom of choice that nearly always accompanies any new reproductive technology, but also, in this case, by the evolving meanings of sex selective ART, which seemed to so neatly categorize as "Western," coded as being individually determined, being gender neutral, producing desired babies, and supporting "family balance." It became clear that a discursive shift was occurring, displacing "sex selection" as a signifier of these practices. Clinicians, bioethicists, self-help authors, and users increasingly used *gender* in place of *sex*, and sometimes avoided the term *selection* entirely. For example, as the scientific director of the MicroSort clinical trial explained to me, "When one hears the term *sex selection*, there is a knee-jerk reaction that it is discriminatory against women . . . I think *gender* is a more palatable word for many people in the US" (IF [interview file] 12/8/10–12/22/10). A MicroSort advertisement appearing in the *New York Times* Sunday Styles section in the summer of 2003 exclusively used *gender* and *gender selection*, but the director stressed that in scientific publications and in conversations with the FDA, GIVF scientists used *sex selection*, which he acknowledged was the more accurate term.

Although I recall hearing a bemused fellow activist ridicule the inaccuracy of "gender" selection, I myself was not always so sure. As a scholar in a field where these terms have profound implication, I recognized the ways in which sex selective ART challenged the idea of sex as a preordained trait. Anthropologists Tine Gammeltoft and Ayo Wahlberg distinguish selective reproductive technologies from assisted reproductive technologies as practices that guide rather than assist nature. As such, sex selective ART challenges the idea that the sex composition of our children must be left to fate (Gammelthoft and Wahlberg 2014). These technologies certainly hold the potential to denaturalize sex, giving humans the ultimate

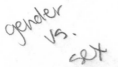

ability to select biologies and thereby identities, subjectivities, and destinies. Yet, we know that the real world makes this possibility contingent upon social and cultural power dynamics and inequalities. The dimensions of race and nation are increasingly difficult to ignore, begging an intersectional analysis of sex selection that can study the impact of these practices beyond sex and gender alone.

I have argued elsewhere that although sex has increasingly become biomedically alterable (within the confines of the female/male binary), gender remains overdetermined by body geography. Consumers of sex selective ART seek to choose the sex of sperm or embryos on the basis of an imagined already gendered child. While the use of sex selective ART does not necessarily foreclose raising children in non-normative gendered ways, anecdotes in popular media suggest that gender expectations and desires of parents are fueled by normative gender stereotypes. Typically we hear about racially unmarked "American" women longing for girls with whom they can go shopping and paint fingernails (Steel 2003, Belkin 1999, Thompson 2004). Perhaps what parents really aim to select *is* a cis form of gender. In effect, consumers choose the sex of babies as a guarantee of child gender, thereby re-affixing gender to sex, a connection that feminist theorists have long sought to unravel.

Early feminist theorists like Gayle Rubin constructed a liberatory version of a sex/gender binary in order to oppose arguments that related women's oppression to a fixed biological destiny of females and to highlight the social construction of gender (Rubin [1975] 1997). Discourses around sex selective ART, however, reinforce the idea of sex as a foundational category of gender, because the choice between blue and pink ultimately translates to the chromosomal options of either XX or XY. Sex selection seems to lock in or fuse societal or parental gender expectations and desires at the site of the sexed infant body, fetus, embryo, or sex chromosome of sorted sperm. In this way, sex selection renaturalizes gender in sex. Rather than sex determining gender, these practices reorder gender *before* sex. They add fodder to the questioning of the sex/gender distinction by Judith Butler, Anne Fausto-Sterling, and other feminist theorists since the 1990s, who direct us to recognize the myriad ways in which sex is simultaneously both a material *and* a social construction.

In changing the name of the practice, physician/entrepreneurs, patient/ consumers, ethicists, and others vested in the emerging practice insisted on its essential difference from non-Western practices of sex selection, which they coded as culturally determined, gender biased, wrongful, and causing population imbalance in sex ratio. That is, they insisted that the developing practice of sex selective ART was unlike sex selective abortion. Yet, within a globalized market, the desire to select sex voiced by those who can afford ART is increasingly interpreted as "Western" regardless of the cultural context or global region from which those desires originate. Are these sex selective ART practices essentially the same as or different from sex selective abortion? The answer turns out to be not so simple.

In this book, I have chosen to name sex selective practices that have evolved around a use of MicroSort and/or PGD in combination with ARTs "lifestyle sex selection." *Lifestyle sex selection* is comparable to *social* or *nonmedical sex selection*, terms used to indicate practices not applied toward disease prevention. Implicated in the technoscientific practices I investigate are, of course, multiple other forms of selection beyond sex alone to ensure the birth of an able-bodied child. Disability studies scholars Anita Ghai (2002) and Adrienne Asch (1999) remind us that what we classify as medical and nonmedical has implications for what we all view as lives worth birthing and living. In this book I use the dominant distinction made by reproductive medicine professionals and bioethicists between medical and nonmedical sex selection precisely to show the expansion of medical jurisdiction into an area of life that no longer needs to be redefined as pathological. As *biomedicalized* interventions, MicroSort and PGD fulfill a need based on a lifestyle desire to transform parental and family identity and constitution.

By retaining *sex* and *selection* in this naming, I am in some ways claiming sameness over difference, insisting not only on a common moral and ethical standard for (sex selective) ART *and* abortion but also on a critical feminist interpretation that is inclusive of both. While the book clearly focuses on the emerging practice of sex selective ART, I have kept the biopolitical contexts that gave rise to sex selective abortion globally in close view throughout. By appending *lifestyle*, however, I do acknowledge difference—the difference that these practices make in a global biopolitical and moral economy of reproduction. *Lifestyle sex selection* denotes a practice of imagining one's future self and family contingent upon the sex of future offspring and trying to realize that dream using technoscientific means. Constituted as benign and devoid of gender bias in a hierarchy of

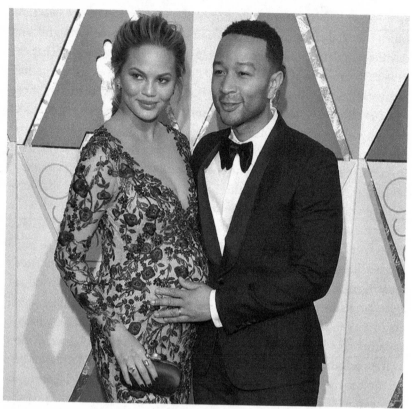

I.1. Stock image of Chrissy Teigen and John Legend reproduced in a *Self* magazine article on their use of sex selective PGD (Miller 2016)

global sex selection practices, the practice runs parallel to other processes of biomedicalization that have since 1985 expanded medical jurisdiction to lifestyle wishes. American popular culture figures Chrissy Teigen (model) and John Legend (musician) made headlines in 2016 for their use of PGD to select a girl. In an interview with *People Magazine*, Teigen expresses this desire: "I think I was most excited and allured by the fact that John would be the best father to a little girl. That excited me," she said. "It excited me to see . . . just the thought of seeing him with a little girl. I think he deserves a little girl. I think he deserves that bond" (Kast 2016; figure I.1).

Teigen imagines Legend in a paternal role that is not only "best" or most effective "with a little girl," but also most happy. She describes him as entitled to experiencing "that bond." Indeed, among issues concerning life itself, the moral imperative to be healthy includes an imperative to be happy. The idea that the gender composition of children is an important element of the heteronormative family ideal in the West is not new, even if lifestyle sex selection is. In the 1950 movie *Tea for Two*, for example, actress Doris Day proposes in song to her beau a future hetero-romance in which the vision of happiness is connected to their making a small, two-child family with "balanced" gender composition. The song further suggests that a relational gender preference of a son or daughter may be particularly desired by either the father or mother and is part of that imagined happiness.[2]

## The Representational and Structural Strategies Constitutive of Lifestyle Sex Selection

Like many who write about mechanisms that drive global forms of inequality with respect to the regimes of internationalized development and global capital, I rely on recognizable but imperfect terms that differentiate geopolitically between the privileged rich and marginalized poor (Mohanty 2003, 539). Most recognized among these are "global North" and "global South," their antecedents, "First World" and "Third World," and "the West and the Rest." During the heyday of the "global population crisis" that elicited fears of a "population explosion" in the latter half of the twentieth century, these categories marked peoples and areas as sites of intervention for population control. Today these terms may seem out of touch with contemporary public discourse that refers to countries such as India and China as "rising" superpowers with globally competitive economic and military might rather than underdeveloped (Schake and Manuel 2016, Ikenberry 2008). Despite the shifting political-economic reality of "rising Asia," I want to highlight the persistence of such Orientalist strategies to maintain inequality between what cultural studies scholar Stuart Hall (2006) calls "the West and the Rest." Orientalism is "the way in which the Orient has been represented in Europe through an imaginative geography that divides East and West, confirming Western superiority and enabling, if not actually constituting, European domination of those negatively portrayed regions known as 'East'" (Abu-Lughod [2001] 2013, 218). Hall claims that Orientalist discourse remains relevant beyond the study of historical imperialist strategies:

This discourse continues to inflect the language of the West, its image of itself and "others," its sense of us and them, its practices and relations of power towards the Rest. It is especially important for the languages of racial inferiority and ethnic superiority which still operate so powerfully across the globe today. So, far from being a "formation" of the past and only of historical interest, the discourse of "the West and the Rest" is alive and well in the modern world. (2006, 173)

Not only do Orientalist strategies remain relevant today, but the "imagined geographies" of the West and non-West have become ever more flexible cultural formations that can dislodge from their referential geographic sites to travel and recontextualize (Ong 1999, Grewal 2005). The West can locate in "rising Asia" just as much as the non-West can locate in the US or Europe.

Furthermore, cultural formations interrelate with politics and economy. Describing a US domestic context, feminist sociologist Laura Mamo explains that the effects of neoliberalism in late capitalism include "cultural wars that rhetorically ensure the false separation of culture from economic issues" *and* a "multicultural equality politics that effaces inequality" (2010, 176). I argue that the same effects apply globally in the case of lifestyle sex selection. To rhetorically challenge the "false separation" between culture and the economy, I refer to two overlapping "cultural-economic" assemblages at work in the constitution of lifestyle sex selection: the cultural economy of Orientialism and of multiculturalism.

The transition of sex selective ART from an ethically controversial to an ethically ambivalent practice relied on an Orientalist strategy that condemns sex selective abortion as essentially other, inferior, and tied culturally to the East, or Asian regions of the world. It produced a cultural formation based on race/ethnicity that is rooted in the neocolonizing international population and development regimes that maintained a divide between nations of the West and the non-West in the latter half of the twentieth century. It is a boundary-making project that creates hierarchical differences between people and contexts.

At the same time, the viability of sex selective ART as a market relies on rising affluence in many parts of the non-Western world as well as globalized market channels that enable service provision across borders. It produces a "multicultural equality" formation based on class that roots in the neoliberal regimes of globalization. It is a boundary-breaking project constitutive of sameness between people and contexts that masks inequality.

As Clarke et al. argue, "Context matters, not as a unidirectional cause but as situated, constitutive conditions of the techno-social shaping of meanings and practices" (2010, ix). While I begin with a local "Western-" and US-framed iteration of sex selective ART, my approach shows how this seemingly *discrete, bounded national practice* involves "techno-social shaping," which makes boundaries of contrast to other biopolitical "sites" of sex selection, especially within contexts of population control in the global non-West. As such, I conceptualize lifestyle sex selection as a *continuously global site* in a Saidian figurative sense of contrast to "other," wrongful forms and sites of sex selection. At the same time, the actual practices of lifestyle sex selection involve boundary crossings to extend into the increasingly transnational reproductive economy of Fertility Inc., quite literally practiced across geopolitical divides, involving not only multiple nation-states but also multiple and enmeshed transnational consumer cultures.

In this book, I explore how lifestyle sex selection constitutes a Western formation even though (or perhaps precisely because) many Western countries such as Canada and those in Europe formally condemn all forms of sex selection as unethical, and non-Western peoples with financial capital seek ART for sex selective purposes. I aim to show that "the West and the Rest" distinction remains powerful to this case precisely because it can sustain these apparent contradictions.

In addition to representational strategies, economic and political shifts create the structural conditions and mechanisms by which lifestyle sex selection operates. The practice situates within the increasingly transnational market operations of Fertility Inc. Dubbed "cross-border reproductive care" by the profession, the multinationally networked operations of fertility clinics and laboratories not only create mechanisms for market transactions across borders but also make up the institutional means to decenter state authority in the governance of reproductive technologies. Decentering state authority is further reinforced by the increasing localization and retreat from the international sphere of women's health and reproductive justice movements as they face challenges from right-wing political elements at home. The prospect of appealing to the state for the centralized collection of data on sex selection and regulation of reproductive markets becomes untenable when government mechanisms and the issue of sex selection are increasingly politically hijacked by anti-abortion movements that profess gender equality concerns in their bid to restrict abortion access and rights.

## The Importance of Destabilizing Reproductive Binaries

Lifestyle sex selection provides me with a key optic through which to theorize how pro- and anti-natalism are both part of the same integrated processes that create and sustain stratified reproduction. While this insight is not new, feminist theory on reproductive technologies sometimes falls into the trap of binaried logics (see figure I.2). Through a narrow focus on singular technologies and localized contexts, it is easy to pigeonhole reproductive technology users into rigid strata that correlate to one side or the other of these dichotomies.

| **I.2  Dichotomized World of Reproductive Technologies** |
|---|
| **valued**/despised reproduction |
| **conceptive**/contraceptive |
| **wealthy**/poor |
| **white**/ people of color |
| **rational**/irrational |
| **(in)fertility**/(over)fertility |
| **developed West**/developing non-West |
| **individuals**/populations |
| **medicalization**/population control |

Within a globalizing reproductive market, however, the category of valued reproduction, for example, does not simply correlate to a whole category of people (such as those that are wealthy or racialized white, etc.), or to a set of (conceptive) technologies, or to a world region (e.g., the developed West). New kinds of biovalue have emerged through the possibility of reproductive exchange (such as through gamete selling and "renting wombs") or in the construction of an active biocitizen—a "prudent yet enterprising individual, actively shaping his or her life course through acts of choice" (Rose and Novas 2005, 458) who participates as consumer in a "political economy of hope" (458). There are multiple new ways in which reproductive processes stratify. What is valued or not (and how) is contingent upon the situated context of reproductive activities within globalized neoliberal state and market structures.

With the development of sex selective ART, two sets of discourses around sex selection emerged that correspond to either side of these fault lines (see figure I.3). The divide promotes facile ideas about cultural difference that maintain a rigid divide between the West and the Rest, and by extension between the meanings of sex selective ART and sex selective abortion. This rift obfuscates the co-construction (and co-implication) of transnational technological practices and cross-cultural changes in society wrought by globalization and late capitalism. It leaves unchallenged a dominant narrative of sex selective ART as an unbiased Western practice of sex selection that balances families and meets individual women's desires. Relying on assumptions of cultural difference, the narrative dangerously re-stigmatizes abortion within a context where abortion rights remain fragile and anti-abortion strategies ingenuously deploy the issue of sex selection as a rationale for policy that can potentially curb abortion access through racial profiling.

| **I.3   Sex Selective ART/Sex Selective Abortion** |
|---|
| **Western**/non-Western<br>**individually determined**/culturally determined<br>**unbiased**/backward<br>***desired babies***/missing girls<br>**family balance**/population imbalance |

In this book, I argue that an increasingly stratified global system of sex selection requires a feminist critique that actively conjoins normally separated biopolitical spheres. Situated reproductive practices since 1995, especially those involving border crossings, occur in increasingly enmeshed transnational and biopolitical contexts that require feminist theoretical frames to actively breach a dichotomous world of reproductive technology. With a vast offering of technological innovations and practices, the transnational reproductive economy elicits circuits of traveling electronic communications, regulatory forms, ethical principles, clinicians, brokers, equipment, technologies, body parts, patients, and donors. Within this marketplace, multiple biopolitical and cultural influences become increasingly entangled, and dichotomized ways of thinking about the contexts of reproductive technology use across global and local divides fail to capture the reinforcement or production of new inequalities.

A few feminist theorists of reproduction have perceived the importance of converging frames. For example, anthropologist Marcia Inhorn, in her study of a "quest for conception" within the pervasive anti-natal context of Egypt in the late twentieth century, explained that "fertility and infertility exist in a dialectical relationship of contrast, such that the understanding of one leads to a much greater understanding of the other" (1994, 23). More recently, historian Michelle Murphy, drawing on Achille Mbembe (2003) and others, asserted that Foucault's notion of biopolitics "also always involved necropolitics—distributions of death effects and precariousness—at the same time as it could foster life" (2012, 13). Murphy proposed approaching biopolitics as a "topology" that can account for "(1) multiplicity, (2) uneven spatiality, and (3) entanglements" in order to make explicit linkages between feminist health movement practices in California in the 1970s, national public health, and international population control programs (12–13). Both authors intentionally link seemingly discrepant phenomena. Inhorn looks at the experience of infertility in the context of "overpopulation"; Murphy compares what she calls the "protocols" of 1970s local US feminist self-help clinics with those of fertility clinics engaged in population control efforts in Bangladesh and other parts of the world.

Dorothy Roberts also makes the case for the importance of converging frames as seen through the evolution of her thinking on race and reproduction. Her initial theorizing at times tended to fortify reproductive dualisms: "Racial injustice infects the use of new reproductive technologies no less than it infects the use of birth control. While too much fertility is seen as a Black woman's problem to be curbed through welfare policy, too little fertility is seen as a white woman's problem to be cured through high-tech interventions. The new reproduction is designed for the creation of white babies" (1997, 292). In more recent work, however, Roberts rethinks this relationship. "In the last several years. . . . I have come to reconsider once again the opposition of white women and women of color in the reproductive caste system," she writes. "A reproductive dystopia for the twenty-first century could no longer exclude women of color from the market for high-tech reprogenetics. Rather, it would take place in a society in which racial and economic divisions are reinforced by the genetic testing extended to them" (2009, 785, 799). As Roberts suggests, a conceptual frame for contemporary reproductive technology practices must account for the growing inclusion of women of color in a range of ART and "reprogenetic" practices.

While several feminist scholars have perceived a need for analysis attentive to convergent biopolitical frames, feminist law scholar Lisa Ikemoto provides a particularly illuminating example. Ikemoto unpacks undercurrents of meaning not visible in dominant narratives that entitle purchasers to reproductive services, even those services whose very obtainability depends on the existence of prevailing inequalities (she refers mainly to surrogacy and egg donation accessed across differences in wealth between poorer and richer nations). The "family formation" narrative centers the "yearning" of infertile couples willing to travel across the world for children, and the "free market" narrative views third parties in ART as "free agents." She considers how the long-standing narrative of population control fuses with the other two to support the "sense of entitlement" to purchase services via "reproductive tourism."

> Both narratives [family formation and free market] express a sense of entitlement. Purchaser's power may account for some of that. Yet, the claim to purchaser's power here is not based solely on greater wealth. The use of women for their biological capacity to reproduce, in a context in which geopolitical differences between departure points and destination spots often account for the wealth disparities, supports a sense of entitlement. In addition, well established narratives that describe low-income women, women of color, and women in less developed nations as "too fertile" nourish the claim of the infertile to ART use as their due. In other words, the identity of those who provide eggs and gestation for others overlaps with those deemed in need of population control. The population control narrative has already cast the women sought for eggs and surrogacy as subalterns. In doing so, the population control narrative has prepared the ground for claims of entitlement in the family formation and market narratives. (Ikemoto 2009, 307)

Ikemoto traces how preexisting ideas about differentially valued reproduction of peoples around the world (constituted through a narrative of population control) contribute to emerging global forms and assemblages in "reproduction tourism." In a similar way, I seek to reveal the implicit workings of a population control narrative in lifestyle sex selection so that I can apprehend the dynamic form of inequality erased by the dominant narrative of family balancing.

How do the meanings of ARTs or pro-natalist technologies configure in relation to abortion and anti-natal ones? As women's, gender, and sexuality studies (WGS) scholar Laura Briggs reflects, "The politics of abortion haunts the reproductive technology clinic" (2010, 366). Focusing on those ghosts, dislocations (cultural and other kinds), and bio-necro-political entanglements can productively destabilize both taken-for-granted notions that sex selection practices are culturally and spatially bound (Narayan 1997) and the presumed sex selective ART/abortion contrast that sustains a globally stratified system of sex selection. Below I review how three key reproductive binaries—individual/social, medicalization/population control, and pro-/anti-natal technology—influenced interpretations of sex selection in feminist literature. In each case, I show the evolution of these conversations as they arrived at a point of impasse beyond which I am seeking to move the analysis. I point out discrepant principles or metholodologies and a lack of concepts that in my view have stalled feminist analysis on sex selection.

## Individual (rights)/Social (justice)

Feminist perspectives on sex selection entered the academic literature in the 1980s within texts on "new reproductive technologies," or "NRTs," which at the time included IVF and prenatal diagnostic technologies.[3] Janice Raymond led one of the earliest discussions, stemming from a conference held in 1979 at Hampshire College (1981). Gena Corea et al.'s (1985) *Man-Made Women* devotes four out of seven chapters to the topic. These theorists viewed preconception forms of sperm separation and prenatal diagnostic technologies and their potential use for selective abortion alongside IVF as "new" technological practices that portended the increasing medicalization of women's reproduction, loss of control by women in reproductive technological processes, and loss of women themselves. As

Raymond recalls from the 1979 sessions on the topic, "Women had listened to several days of how we have been victimized by a whole spectrum of reproductive technologies, from contraception to sterilization abuse. Yet the impinging reality of sex preselection moved our discussion of manipulative medical technologies into the realm of *previctimization*, i.e., the spectre of women being destroyed and sacrificed before even being born" (1981, 177).

Mary Anne Warren's 1985 book, *Gendercide: The Implications of Sex Selection*, steered the direction of another set of writings that relied on philosophical concepts on ethics, weighing arguments in favor of or condemning sex selection on consequentialist (potential to cause harm) or nonconsequentialist (principled) grounds. Warren saw no difference on moral grounds between "early sex-selective abortion" and "preconceptive sex selection," judging as "rational" or "altruistic" even those sex selective decisions made under the constraints of structural dimensions of patriarchy, such as choosing sons because they could inherit or because they would not have to face gender-based discrimination (83–85). Canadian feminist philosopher Christine Overall disagreed: "Granted, it may be kinder on an individual basis to avoid producing daughters who will suffer grievous injury through nutritional deprivation, genital mutilation, sexual abuse, exploitative labour, and dangerous procreation. But choosing sons for that reason is still a way of saying yes, however obscurely or reluctantly, to patriarchal power and the oppression of women" (1987, 687).

Although the philosophical debate on the morality of sex selection continued, most of these North American writers agreed that outright prohibitions of the practice might unduly impinge upon civil liberties, specifically the right to abortion (Warren 1985, Wertz and Fletcher in Holmes and Purdy 1992, Holmes in Callahan 1995). Referring to their own perspectives as "feminist," and in conversation with one another, their work reveals a central tension between the individual and the social. Rosalind Petchesky grappled with that tension in her classic text *Abortion and Woman's Choice*. How do feminists reconcile an individual's desire for a specifically sexed child with the social need of ensuring equality between the sexes? Petchesky, who sided with the individual in multiple cases in which a woman's desires or needs were pitted against social ones, made one surprising exception. She soundly denounced sex selection as "grossly sexist and therefore antifeminist and immoral," regardless of whether the decision involved choosing against a male or female ([1984] 1990, 349). This illustrates, per Petchesky, that "'a woman's right to control her body' is not absolute" (7).

During the 1990s through advancement of the idea of reproductive justice (RJ), women of color scholars and activists in the US addressed the individual/social tension by correcting notions of reproductive rights overdetermined by libertarian, abortion-centric, and market-driven notions of individual choice. Silliman et al. (2002), in *Policing the National Body*, for example, highlighted a broader range of issues emerging in the 1990s such as the criminalization of pregnant, drug-using women as well as welfare and immigration controls, alongside the ongoing issues of coercive contraception and sterilization abuse that had played a role in motivating the population policy reform agenda at the ICPD. RJ movements in the US drew on the insights of critical race theory to account for multiple and intersecting oppressions, foregrounding notions of justice based on the social and political recognition of marginalized persons (Silliman et al. 2004, Luna and Luker 2013, ACRJ 2005).

Yet, as I will discuss in chapter 4, the normative call for reproductive justice only appears to prioritize social issues over individual ones. A radical transformation in the reproductive justice agenda on sex selection in the US reveals how integrated rights and justice claims produce multiple kinds of "individuals" and "socials" that do not necessarily oppose each other. It is not just that social needs should rank as equal to individual rights, or that individual rights claims ought not be made at the expense of the oppression of marginalized communities. Reproductive justice claims on the issue of sex selection in the US demonstrate that individual rights claims can be instrumentalized in the name of social justice to advance the social and political recognition of those who are marginalized.

## Medicalization/Population Control

One distinguishing feature of writing on NRTs was an overarching commitment to explore "reproductive control over women" in a variety of global settings, but some of these theorists imagined that forms of control—whether medicalization or population control—differed based upon the geopolitical context. For example, Raymond argues:

The production of fertility and infertility, that is, the ways in which both are created and commodified as medical problems, is very much linked with the production of distinctively different technologies developed for use in different parts of the world. The ideology of infertility in the West is based on a double standard. Children who are technologically conceived at high cost in the industrialized world—a staggering cost to women's well-being and a high economic cost—are the potential children whose conception is thwarted in the Third World, through sterilization, harmful contraceptives, and sex predetermination, not to mention the existing children who die of poverty, malnutrition and other causes. Keeping First-Third World connections in view enables us not to lose sight of the global picture of technological reproduction. (1993, 2)

Raymond's assumption that "different technologies" function as mechanisms of control in "different parts of the world" cements both the ART/sterilization binary and the divide between forms of social control (medicalization/population control) on global West/Rest lines. Today, reproductive practices involving transnational exchanges of ova, surrogacy, cross-bordered, and cross-cultural uses of ARTs compel a return to "the global" for reasons other than (but not exclusive of) the desire to ensure that "the well-being of one set of people and one set of women is not based on and paid for by the exploitation and degradation of another set of people and another set of women" (Mies 1991, 34). Today a transnational focus requires questioning an implied divide in classic feminist theorizations of NRTs between medicalization as a form of social control for women in the developed world and population control for women in developing regions. Not only do these two processes coalesce in the development of lifestyle sex selection, but feminist theorists perceived a need for their updating in light of major social-technical, political, cultural, and economic changes under way in late capitalism that fundamentally impact how the regimes of medicine and population control operate.

In their original article on biomedicalization, later expanded to a book, Clarke and her coauthors (2003) identified a need to expand on Irving Zola's approach to medicine as an institution of social control, initially put forth in the 1970s. They argued that the explanatory power of medicalization could not fully account for a late twentieth-century context of new social forms and major changes in the organization of contemporary medicine. They illuminated these changes by outlining politico-economic, technoscientific, and sociocultural processes that together constitute biomedicalization. These processes no longer require the production of illness identities via pathologization. Rather, they simply exist within biomedical contexts and are subsumed by biomedical meanings.

Though the medicalization of sex selection became possible in the late 1970s with the emergence of prenatal diagnostic technologies (PND) such as ultrasound scanning and amniocentesis, which could detect fetal sex, it did not occur. Clearly, the presence of the technological possibility alone was not enough to precipitate the processes of medicalization, even though PND technologies represented a significant scientific advance for their time, just as sex selective ART would nearly two decades later. Although PND technologies powerfully amplified the medical surveillance and women's experience and understandings of pregnancy, when applied toward sex selection within the context of population control, they could not shake the associative meanings of perversion related to uncontrollably fertile, primitive bodies prone to commit "social evil." As awareness of the practice of sex selective abortion grew, the "problem" was defined in social, cultural, political, and demographic, but certainly not medical, terms.

If I assume that just as with sex selective abortion, the emergence of the ART-dependent technologies alone was not sufficient to determine the biomedicalization of sex selection, I must ask, what did? I argue that lifestyle sex selection exemplifies the basic interactive processes of biomedicalization as defined by Clarke et al. Further, I posit a relationship between the nonmedicalization of sex selective abortion and the biomedicalization of sex selective ART. I contend that the powerful factors and processes that continue to prevent the medicalization of sex selection via abortion are integral, indeed constitutive of, the biomedicalization of sex selection via ART.

Ideas about "population control," unlike those about medicalization, did not undergo a major conceptual overhaul. By the early 1990s, ahead of the ICPD in Cairo, feminist theorizations of population control and reproductive rights circulated within both scholarly and policy arenas. They had a strong impact on the events and practices surrounding the ICPD, and they initiated the discourse shift that completely erased "control" within population discourses. Political scientist Paige Whaley Eager, who studied the Cairo "paradigm shift," describes how "the language, assumptions, and norms supporting population control were supplanted by the language, assumptions, and norms supporting reproductive rights and health" (2004, 2). Shifting population discourses, I suggest, may have become increasingly incongruent with shifting medicalization discourses, which have elaborated on but not erased ideas of power and control. Rather than discard or replace medicalization, Clarke et al. redefined the term to account for contemporary contextual shifts. While some analysts have gone so far as to declare population control "history" (Connelly 2003), others have struggled to acknowledge and describe the changes afoot in population control processes without a new term that can simultaneously convey what has stayed the same. Among them, Susanne Schultz interpreted the "speechlessness" on the part of women's NGOs in response to ongoing population control violations and sterilization atrocities in Peru *after* the ICPD as "an example of the transformation of the hegemonic project of international population policies" (2010, 176). Like Mohan Rao and Sarah Sexton (2010), Schultz argues that "the very focus on reproductive health (rather than explicitly on demographic goals) made it possible to reformulate anti-natalist objectives (albeit indirectly) as the management of reproductive risks at the micro level of individual behavior and responsibility for one's self" (177). Schultz conveys how population control processes increasingly work like medicalization, involving the active participation of women users of technology (see also Riessman 1983). Population control mechanisms, then, have hardly disappeared (Hendrixson n.p.), though our ways of naming them may have. They recur both directly and indirectly, sometimes through unrecognizable means.

Clarke et al. describe their case studies as "sites," not necessarily geographical locations, "where we found particular bodies, identities, and corporealities becoming *biomedical* objects for (re)configuration in old and new ways" (2010, ix, emphasis mine). By recognizing lifestyle sex selection as a Foucauldian biopolitical project of disciplining individual bodies and regulating populations, we can see how "particular bodies, identities, and corporealities" become *biopolitical* "objects for (re)configuration in old and new ways." Practices of "making up" individuals or "making up" populations are not unlike, and often work in and through each other (Hacking 1986, Curtis 2001). How do the microphysics of power, individuals, and "regimes of the self" (Rose 2006, 154) work in conjunction with a macrophysics of power, states/markets, populations, and global regimes?

Attention to the interdependence of individuals and populations within "the government of population" may assist in considering how categorizations have both individualizing and totalizing subjective dimensions. Moving away from thinking about population only in terms of "occupants of a national territory," as Bruce Curtis suggests, can reveal such "(re)configurations." Grewal invokes this idea in her discussion of 1990s global discourses on "women's rights as human rights." She explains that the power of the discourse lay in its ability to represent "women" simultaneously as a population and as autonomous individuals "who could become … global citizens; this was the 'third world' victim who had become a global subject" (2005, 130). The invocations of women's reproductive rights in changed population discourses emanating from the 1994 ICPD may function in a similar way. Rethinking population control requires remaining cognizant of what happens to older national and international forms as new deterritorialized forms are constructed alongside them. In the case of sex selection, the figure of a "Third World" victim of a backward, sexist culture does not diminish, but can flexibly transform into a global bio-citizen exercising consumer choice within Fertility Inc. In this way, the constitution of a biomedicalized form of sex selection reinforces the nonmedicalization of sex selective abortion already secured through population control to stratify a global system of sex selection practices.

Feminist scholars have recently renewed the process of collectively identifying the "old maps" and "new terrains" of population control, grappling with how to name the multiple and interrelated ways population control manifests in the contemporary moment.[4] Following the core, overarching analytical characteristic of the interactive processes of biomedicalization, it may be conceptually useful to perceive a shift from *control over* to *transformations of* (in this case, reproductive) phenomena. At the risk of overusing the prefix *bio-*, I argue that the significant theoretical apparatus that has elaborated *bio-* in relation to medicalization, technology, politics, economy, and so forth, has overlooked changes to the international population control order. To that end, I tentatively offer the term *biopopulationism* to convey both what has changed and what has stayed the same in that order. Population control did not simply disappear, but can function without explicit "pathologizing" of fertility and intervention focused solely on reducing population numbers. As Sharmila Rudruppa reminds us, "Continued indiscriminate sterilization of working-class women" geared toward controlling population growth in India resulted in an average of twelve deaths per month through botched sterilizations between 2003 and 2012 (2015, 172). Yet, the regime of population control manifests in new ways that center *bio*, or life itself, rather than strictly population as the object of intervention. Contemporary globalized bio-politics and bioeconomies shift focus away from nation-states toward individuated subjects who manage reproductive risks within markets, not merely for the sake of controlling whether and when to have children, but to transform individual and family identities and the experience of life itself. *Bio-* signifies the ways in which people engage their reproductive bodies toward multiple ends—not merely to have or not have children, but to live particular kinds of lives. The prefix speaks to the lifestyle mani-festation of reproduction through sex selective ART.

I borrow the term *populationism* from Ian Angus and Simon Butler, who use the term "to refer to ideologies that attribute social and ecological ills to human numbers" (2011, xxi). I build upon this definition to discuss not only forms of population control directly focused on human numbers, but also the growing preoccupation with "quality" in family composition, precisely as fertility rates continue their downward trend. From the begin-ning, the promise of selectively producing more valued and desired children by avoiding disability or choosing sex have been integral parts of the same sociotechnical strategies that limit population and family size. Susanne Schultz describes populationist mechanisms that connect "abstract, appar-ently egalitarian, purely quantitative rationales, referring to a homogenous national (or global) population with strategies of classist selection and racist exclusion" (2015, 339). These mechanisms assert notions of human-ity often abstracted in numerical form in relation to abstract notions of nature (or cultures). They then selectively identify sources of relative excess (too many poor, too many immigrants) or scarcity (natural resources, endangered cultures, climates, and environment) (Lohman 2005, Schultz 2015). Thus, beneath the framing of quantitative, apparently apolitical measures such as fertility rates or sex ratios at birth can lurk a population-ist project that identifies the presence and/or reproduction of othered populations as moral problems requiring condemnation, if not social prob-lems in need of control, surveillance, or policing. Biopopulationism dis-tinguishes some "bodies, identities, and corporealities" as rational and others as (morally or environmentally) polluting, thereby constructing (while also stratifying) flexible categories that can be breached to enable transformations between the object of international population control and the subject engaged in biomedical markets.

While the scholars who initially conceptualized biomedicalization focused "almost exclusively on the US case, holding the nation-state relatively constant" (Clarke et al. 2010, 380), my study has taken up their call to pursue the transnational travels of biomedicalization through attention to sex selective ART as a global form and traveling assemblage. I highlight how transnational biomedicalization processes depend on the politics of social location within an old international population order, even as the practices themselves operate across various sites of national belonging both within and across the geopolitically bordered US.

## Pro-/Anti-natalist Reproductive Technologies

To breach the sex selective ART/abortion divide, I face in this project the challenge of weaving together insights drawn from literature that focuses on either pro- or anti-natalist technologies; these bodies of work differ somewhat in their overall theoretical and methodological orientation.

Working at the cross-sites of science and technology studies (STS) and anthropology, scholars tend to treat fertility technologies as cultural objects, illuminating reproduction as a social and cultural process involving multiple subjects and interests rather than an individual act, choice, or right. Following the STS predilection of revealing the mutual constitution of nature and society, scholars exhibit a fascination with the various ways in which "artificial" reproduction via ARTs upended notions of the "natural" or "biological facts" of reproduction (Strathern 1992, Ragoné and Franklin 1998, Thompson 2005). They avoid readings of technologies as deterministic in their influence on society, or potentially dangerous and unsafe in and of themselves. Rather, technologies are understood as "socio-technical products, which are shaped by human and nonhuman factors" (Inhorn and Birenbaum-Carmeli 2008, 178). As a result, these perspectives on ART accord technology a far less negatively deterministic role in their effects on society than earlier critiques of NRTs.

Literature on anti-natal reproductive technology takes a different tack, interpreting NRTs primarily as political objects that are instrumentalized as a means to achieve individual or social control. Having a proclivity for the "global," this literature conceptually engages "population" and "development." It foregrounds and problematizes the contexts of primarily abortion, contraception, and sterilization use, often by women in or of the global non-West. It applies political-economic analysis to the contexts of reproductive technology use, utilizing human rights and social justice discourses to question, refine, and/or elaborate on concepts stemming from foundational feminist theorizations such as "choice," "control," "freedom," and "rights." A majority of perspectives on anti-natalist technologies that raise concerns about the abuses of population control call for meaningful informed consent in reproductive decision making, questioning not the use of particular technologies per se, but rather the assumption that new technologies automatically spell progress or an enhancement of choice for women, as presumed by dominant liberal views of science (Hartmann 1995, Roberts 1997, Silliman and Bhattacharjee 2002, Silliman et al. 2004).

The few feminist voices on sex selection are overwhelmed either by perspectives stemming from the population sciences on sex selective abortion or by professional bioethicists on sex selective ART. Susan Greenhalgh and Jiali Li, for example, begin their study by pointing out the "remarkably few feminist scholars" who write on "the problem of China's missing girls," which results in demographers defining "the terms in which the issue is understood" (1995, 601–602). As a result, depictions of the problem resort to limited understandings of "gender" and "culture," which demographers treat as apolitical and ahistorical "residual variables" (603). Drawing on qualitative, ethnographic, and demographic data from three villages in China, Greenhalgh and Li counter, "We see the gender dimensions of reproductive values not as contemporary manifestations of traditional culture but as something newly constructed out of the residues of the past and the exigencies of contemporary life. Thus, politics, the state, and history, which are missing from the demographic account, take center stage in ours" (606). Other feminist scholars have also insisted on linking the phenomenon of "missing girls" with contemporary, globalized population and economic policies rather than relying solely on explanations of "cultural son preference." They point to upwardly mobile class and newly forming consumerist cultures as opposed to ahistorical notions of "traditional" culture as drivers of sex selective abortion practice (Croll 2000, Mallik 2003, SAMA 2005).

Few feminist theorists have addressed the contemporary phenomena of sex selective ART, and only recently have scholars, especially from the Asian diaspora, begun to incorporate discussion of both sex selective ART and abortion within a single frame by focusing on the experiences of South Asian immigrants (e.g., Puri et al. 2011, Purewal 2010, Jesudason n.d.). In a similar vein I seek to challenge the differential meanings assigned to global practices divided along a West/Rest binary. This requires a study of multiple interrelated technologies as both cultural *and* political objects, and the interweaving of feminist literature that has provided predominantly political-economic insights on anti-natal technologies with sociocultural perspectives on ART.

## Book Structure

This book organizes along an arc that configures the material, discursive, and institutional formations of lifestyle sex selection from the early moments of its anticipation to its incorporation within Fertility Inc., through its extension through global networks, and finally its contestation among various interested groups.

In chapter 1, I employ STS methods of studying "technoscience-in-the-making" by foregrounding and analyzing the biomedicalization processes involved in the anticipation of lifestyle sex selection. I trace the convergent histories of MicroSort and PGD as these technologies shifted from their origins in livestock reproduction to diagnostic tools fulfilling human medical needs and then to elective interventions of lifestyle sex selection. The discussion focuses on the constitution of lifestyle sex selection transnationally in relation to the maintenance of the nonmedicalization of sex selective abortion.

Chapter 2 turns to how MicroSort and PGD became technologies of hopes and dreams as they merged into Fertility Inc. I highlight how the beginning of structural neoliberalization of the "old" international population order occurred alongside assertions of fertility clinic authority and protection of clinic autonomy from state intervention by various stakeholders in the United States. Rather than representing these processes as structural contrasts or ironies, I argue they are part of a continuum of globalizing biopopulationist processes that involve the biopolitical refashioning of subjects—both individuals and populations.

Within a variety of media such as clinic websites, self-help books and blogs, and popular news sources, the appearance and circulation of new terms, categories, figurative language, and visual images construct a discourse that produces the meaning of sex selection in the public imagination as practiced via ART. In this chapter, I further examine the affective economy that arose and the meanings that had to stabilize in the incorporation of lifestyle sex selection within Fertility Inc. I highlight processes that channel individual biopolitical subjects who are racialized white, nationalized Western, and yearning for a girl. This figure is counterposed to an oppressed population of women stemming from a backward, sexist society who are slaves to their culture and tradition. Disaggregated from this whole is the emergent, individuated, non-Western, diasporic subject, or reproductive traveler, who can purchase a trans-Western form of (temporary) biocitizenship in order to share in the biosocial exchange of "gender dreaming" or disappointment.

Chapter 3 traces the extension of lifestyle sex selection into a global market, presenting the practice as a case study of cross-border reproductive practices similar to movements to access egg donation and surrogacy. In cross-border sex selection, the US is situated as both a destination and a departure site within a growing spectrum of traveling practices. The "transnationalization" of clinics (Ikemoto 2009), as well as the establishment of off-shore labs and sites of clinical operations owned and operated by US clinics, has extended these practices into other globally significant hubs such as Mexico. The entire system challenges bioethical frameworks and escapes national and even weaker international regulatory mechanisms through a global form made up of discrete, informal, clinic-to-clinic networks in which clinics act as endpoints of travel by information, biomaterial, equipment, patients, and providers across borders. Documents that treat sex selection as an international problem ignore this structure, producing directives aimed at nation-states within non-Western regions. Escaping scrutiny and accountability for potential harms related to sex selection, fertility clinics can participate in some part of the growing cross-border sex selection markets even when they reside in jurisidictions in which the practice is illegal.

In chapter 4 I reflect on fifteen years of campaigns on the issue of sex selection in the United States since the emergence of sex selective ART practices. Drawing on the voices of reproductive justice scholar/activists as well as a thematic analysis of campaign material, I track and analyze the claims-making processes involved, particularly through contestations of what is known and not known about these practices. In the context of successfully passed sex selective abortion bans in a growing number of US states since 2008, I take stock of the important resistance strategies to racial profiling and policing of abortion access in more recent inflections of these campaigns. In particular, I highlight what is at stake in debates that revolve around the representation of evidence of sex selection occurring in Asian American communities or within particular nation-states as they appear in cross-fired exchanges between various stakeholders such as reproductive justice or anti-abortion groups.

In the conclusion, I elaborate a feminist intersectional perspective on sex selection that culls the interpretive strengths of *stratified reproduction* and *reproductive justice* to move beyond an analysis of sex selection relying on reductive categories of gender and culture that do not account for class, race/ethnicity, nationality, sexuality, ability, and other axes of difference. Classically defined reproductive justice issues, such as sterilization abuse and coercive contraception, do not disappear within this perspective, but lay the ground for shifting forms of population control. My aim is to conceptually capture biopopulationism by apprehending the complex intermingling of the cultural economy of Orientalism with that of multi-culturalism. Biopopulationism involves reproductive activities that people engage in today to achieve multiple ends, not merely to have or to prevent having their own child, but to live particular kinds of lives.

## Background on ART-Dependent Sex Selection

As this book starts with the scientific products MicroSort and PGD, what follows is an explanation of how these technologies work and other information essential to situating their related applications within a global political economy of reproduction. As a set of technologies constitutive of lifestyle sex selection, MicroSort and PGD are more similar than different. They are both examples of "high" science and technology applied before pregnancy. PGD sexes embryos prior to implantation in a women's womb, while MicroSort sexes sperm before conception. PGD is highly accurate at identifying the sex of embryos. MicroSort is less accurate in differentiating X- from Y-bearing sperm, aiming at best to alter probabilities, shifting sperm populations from the normal 50:50 ratio to a higher proportion of sex-desired sperm. Neither can guarantee the birth of a baby, for they rely on the successful use of ART. Since MicroSort can be applied using intra-uterine insemination, while PGD necessitates IVF, MicroSort sidesteps abortion-related politics more than PGD, which must contend with the morally and ethically contentious issue of producing and potentially disposing of human embryos that do not get transferred for pregnancy. When these technologies were first clinically applied within human medicine to avoid genetic disease, scientists touted both for their ability to avoid repeat pregnancy terminations associated with prenatal diagnostic test results that reveal afflicted fetuses. As a cross-use, multipurpose technology, PGD maintains an anchor to the larger medicalized context of clinical genetics, while MicroSort widened the ambit of clinical indications for sex selection by defining a nonmedical use that came to be called *family balancing*. The push and pull of these various factors, their comparative association with ART, and their disassociation with both sex selective abortion and "pseudo-scientific" methods all reinforce the convergence of PGD and MicroSort into a set of alternative, high-tech sex selection technologies.

The MicroSort trial began after the US Department of Agriculture (USDA) granted GIVF an exclusive license to commercialize the method for human use. The USDA had developed the method originally for use in the livestock industry, patenting its method of sperm sexing under the name Beltsville Sperm Sexing Technology. GIVF renamed its human application complete with a registered trademark signifier, "MicroSort®." In scientific literature the method is identified as "flow cytometric separation of DNA-based X or Y enriched sperm samples." It differs and should not be confused with other methods of sperm separation, such as the Ericsson method or those that involve sperm spinning. I use the trade name "Micro-Sort" in this book not only for the sake of simplicity but also because my data all comes from MicroSort providers. Although the method as of 2010 is no longer under exclusive use license, I did not encounter the method in the field under a different name or provided by any entity other than GIVF or GIVF-recognized ART providers who transact with GIVF-owned labs for sperm sorting.

In 1993, the institutional review board (IRB) at Inova Fairfax Hospital approved the clinical trial only for the indication of sex-linked disease. Two years later, GIVF established its own in-house IRB, which assumed oversight of the trial and approved the extension of MicroSort applications to the "indication" of "family balancing" (Wadman 2001, 178). In the late 1990s, the US Food and Drug Administration (FDA) extended its authority over the clinical trial—to oversee the trial process and make the ultimate determination on MicroSort safety and efficacy.[5] The trial history, thus, divides into two periods: from 1993 to 2000 (GIVF oversight) and from 2000 to 2012 (FDA oversight) (IF 12/8/10–12/22/10).

In the middle of 2008 the trial officially concluded when it reached its sample size limit of 1,050 babies. MicroSort continued to enroll subjects under an FDA policy of "continued access," for which GIVF had to reapply every six months. Meanwhile, while waiting for an FDA determination on the method's safety and efficacy, GIVF began to open MicroSort labs outside of FDA jurisdiction, first in Mexico in 2009. In the summer of 2010, in response to GIVF's fifth application for "continued access," the FDA denied it specifically for the "indication" of "family balancing." Thereafter, MicroSort was available in the US for the medical indication of avoiding X-linked disease only, until GIVF decided in the spring of 2012 to withdraw its application for pre-market approval from the FDA, citing "high costs and regulatory burdens" (IF 12/8/10–12/22/10; Dondorp et al. 2013, 1449). Today, MicroSort sperm sorting takes place only outside the US, but some US clinics agree to receive and use shipped frozen sorted samples of sperm in IVF treatments for their patients.

Although the most important instrument involved in the MicroSort process is the *flow cytometer*, MicroSort should not be understood as an instrument or machine itself, but rather as a process or series of steps that act on the raw material of human sperm. Often contrasted to their earlier kin, the microscope, which permits analysis of a single cell or particle, flow cytometers use a system of cells flowing in a liquid in single file past an optical analysis point, allowing measurement and collection of information on a whole population of cells. Flow cytometers can count and sort cells. Starting with a raw semen sample, lab technicians begin a multistep process of washing and evaluating sperm volume, concentration, motility, and viability before the "specimen is handed off" for staining, which binds to the DNA in the sperm (IF 12/8/10–12/22/10). The "input" sample flows through the cytometer and hits a laser beam, which causes the stain to fluoresce. A detector reads the amount of fluorescence at the sperm's edge to determine if the sperm is oriented correctly. Most are not oriented correctly, do not get read, and are wasted, resulting in far fewer sperm numbers (200,000–400,000) than in the original sample (20–40 million). If the sperm is oriented correctly, another detector reads the fluorescence intensity on the face of the sperm head. Since X sperm have more DNA, they will fluoresce more brightly. Sperm cells with higher intensity fluorescence, for example, will be given a positive charge and then deflected by a negatively charged plate to an "X sort" tube (Schulman and Karabinus 2005, 112; FN [fieldnotes] 9/10/10). This is the basic mechanism by which MicroSort separates X- from Y-bearing sperm populations. Due to the material factors of human sperm that I discuss in chapter 2, MicroSort produces X-based sperm samples of higher purity by about thirteen percentage points than Y-based samples. The technique is therefore more effective at producing girls (Karabinus et al. 2014).

Unlike MicroSort, PGD did not undergo a federally regulated clinical trial and remains largely unregulated by federal mechanisms in the US. The technique was developed in the UK alongside IVF. In the scientific literature, a distinction is sometimes made between preimplantation screening (PGS) and preimplantation genetic diagnosis (PGD). Screening refers to both sex selection and aneuploidy (abnormal chromosome number) screening protocols that do not technically diagnose a disease. However, lay publics such as online self-help communities, journalists of news and popular media, and even many providers drop this distinction and refer to all applications as "PGD," which I also use. PGD is a subset of processes within IVF, taking place after the creation of embryos in the laboratory and before transfer of those embryos back to the women intending to get pregnant. PGD testing often combines sex selection applications with those used to identify some of the main aberrations in chromosome numbers, other kinds of chromosome disorders, or single-gene disorders. PGD involves two major sets of procedures. First developed in the late 1960s, the first procedure is an embryo biopsy, which involves removing a cell from each of the embryos created in the IVF cycle. The second procedure applies a test used to analyze the chromosomal and genetic information contained in the nucleus of the removed cell. For many years after their inception, two main tests yielded information from the cell nuclei removed via embryo biopsy: polymerase chain reaction (PCR) and fluorescence in situ hybridization (FISH), which were both developed during the 1980s. The first clinical application of PGD occurred with PCR, but

FISH served as the test of choice in basic sex selection protocols until about 2009, when a third type of screening procedure, array comparative genomic hybridization (CGH), which tests all twenty-three chromosome pairs, emerged (Fishel et al. 2009).

Inside the cell nucleus, chromosomes are the larger packages that hold DNA. FISH involves first developing a probe, which is a small, unique subsection of DNA molecules that fluoresces, and then allowing that fluorescent probe to bind to its counterpart on a DNA strand that has been unraveled from the helix. Genetic labs sold convenient 2-probe, 5-probe, or 9- and 10-probe kits to ART clinics that had the laboratories and expertise to conduct FISH in-house. Simple chromosomal sex differentiation via FISH requires only two probes, but since sex selection is often enveloped within larger aneuploidy screening protocols, more probes were often used. A 5-probe kit, for example, screened not only for the two sex chromosomes, X and Y, but for chromosomes 13, 18, and 21 because the presence of more than the normal pair, or *too many*, of these chromosomes represents some of the most common "birth defects." Today, advanced DNA analytics improve some of limitations of FISH by allowing a simultaneous screening of all twenty-three chromosome pairs, but these procedures are less likely to occur in-house at IVF clinics.

When I began researching sex selective ART in 2010, PGD protocols typically involved retrieving eggs from a patient's ovaries, fertilizing them, biopsying cells from the resulting embryos after three days, conducting FISH on the biopsied cell, and making decisions about which embryos to transfer back to a patient's uterus after five days based on the PGD results. Five years later, one clinic director described FISH as a "dinosaur" (IF 5/29/15). With the newer molecular tools used in PGD analysis, biopsy and embryo transfer protocols have shifted later. In addition, improved cryopreservation techniques for embryos permit the staggering of IVF cycles and a longer break of time between egg retrieval and embryo transfer. These technological and procedural changes impact the global reproductive market for sex selection by making information about sex now an integrated aspect of PGD analysis, so that all applications of PGD are potentially sex selective, and by creating new kinds of contingencies for traveling patients.

# 1

# From Selecting Sexed Sperm and Embryos to Anticipating Lifestyle Sex Selection

SEX SELECTIVE ART COMPRISES A SET OF TECHNOLOGIES, MICROSORT and PGD, which developed historically on distinct paths, but began to converge as a set of related practices through two major historic turns. The first turn occurred as the technologies crossed from their development within agricultural industry research in the UK and US into the realm of human medicine in the early to mid-1990s. The potential for human applications could not sustain the development of these technologies initially, and in this transfer to human medicine both technologies underwent a process of redefinition—transforming from the endpoint of sex selection (specifically for industrially valued female livestock) to a means of avoiding sex-linked disease. PGD led this transformation and MicroSort piggybacked onto this process of medicalization, defining itself as an adjunct technology to PGD to increase the production of medically needed female human embryos, which may carry but do not express X-linked genetic disease.

A short while later the technologies underwent another process of redefinition as they moved from therapeutic to lifestyle medicine. Defined by Gilbert et al. (2000), lifestyle medicine treats "non-health problems" or "conditions that lie at the boundary between a health need and a lifestyle wish" (1341). In this second transformation, MicroSort led the way by first defining *family balancing*, the desire for a boy or girl to offset an imbalance in the sex of offspring, as an indication for its use. As the technologies shifted from serving as diagnostic tools fulfilling medical needs to elective interventions, their meanings had to stabilize. Together, they became "high-tech gender selection" and formed a new set of sex selection practices with a stake in the biomedical worlds of Fertility Inc.

Paul Rabinow's ethnographic study of polymerase chain reaction (PCR), one of the scientific techniques that appears in this story as a mode of detecting sex for PGD, describes it as "a tool that has the power to create new situations for its use and new subjects to use it" (Rabinow 1996, 7). One of the situations that emerged through a use of PCR is contemporary lifestyle sex selection. The material assemblage of each technology to sex sperm (MicroSort) or sex embryos (PGD) took place for reasons other than human lifestyle sex selection. Yet, their parallel development and medicalization set the stage for their later convergence into a set of tools for lifestyle medicine. Through successive historical turns, the technologies became entwined in processes of first classic medicalization and then biomedicalization.

As medicalized interventions, MicroSort and PGD fulfilled a need linked to reducing or eliminating the risk of disease affliction, which is based on a professional diagnosis. They extended control over pregnancy and reproduction first enabled *during* pregnancy through prenatal diagnostic technologies (PND) to *before* pregnancy. From amniocentesis and chorionic villus sampling to ultrasound and now maternal serum screening—various forms of PND have become routine aspects of prenatal care since the 1970s. These technologies were enrolled in broader processes that pathologized and medicalized pregnancy. When combined with abortion technologies, PND provided a means to avoid having children with chromosomal disorders or genetic mutations resulting in disease. In this sense, the precedence of PND provided a context of *association* for PGD as well as common material-technological modes of analysis (e.g., fluorescence in situ hybridization [FISH] for the detection of specific chromosomes). At the time when reproductive scientists first considered the prospect of a *preimplantation* form of genetic diagnosis, they did not draw a sharp boundary between technologies applied before or during pregnancy, considering them on a continuum of access points where diagnostic results have varying implications. Yet, when the very prospect of developing PGD rested on public advocacy highlighting its ability to avoid abortion, a wedge was driven between genetic selective abortion and genetic selective ART. Insofar as PND raises the potential of abortion depending on results, PND represents a context of *disassociation* for the technologies of lifestyle sex selection.

As *biomedicalized* interventions, MicroSort and PGD fulfill a need based on a lifestyle desire, to transform parental and family identity and constitution. As sociologist Laura Mamo explains, biomedicalization refers to processes in which "there is no longer a prerequisite to pathologize the body to maintain medical authority and jurisidiction; instead biomedicalization extends its reach to include any and all issues concerning life itself, culminating in a moral imperative to be healthy. While cosmetic and other lifestyle issues are already part of U.S. consumer discourse, their place as objects of U.S. biomedicine is intensifying" (2010, 175). This is a story not only of how the technologies developed but also how they became acceptable for lifestyle sex selection. This story is both intertechnological and transnational in scope, and could not be told with a focus on a single technology or local context. I argue that the "techno-social shaping" (Clarke et al. 2010, ix) of lifestyle sex selection took place within a geopolitical configuration of US-UK transatlantic scientific exchange inside Fertility Inc., where biomedicalization processes merged alongside other "high" technologies in the realm of assisted reproduction such as in vitro fertilization (IVF) and intracytoplasmic sperm injection (ICSI). In this case, successful biomedicalization hinged upon the active disassociation by scientists and clinicians of sex selective ART from practices of sex selection that never medicalized, such as "pseudoscientific" preconception interventions, scientific methods involving abortion, or unscientific "low" tech.

In this chapter, I trace the technoscientific history that led to lifestyle applications of sex selective ART through two successive turns and convergences of MicroSort and PGD. While the first turn constituted a process of *medicalization*, the second exemplifies *biomedicalization*. I then situate sex selective ART within a dichotomous world of reproductive technology, exploring the material meanings of MicroSort and PGD in relation to technologies of association or in contrast to the *nonmedicalization* of other technoscientific practices.

## The Development of Sex Selective ART en Route to Lifestyle Sex Selection

In the early 1990s, human clinical trials of both MicroSort and PGD began with the first PGD baby born in 1990 and the first MicroSort baby born in 1995. Both "firsts" involved couples selecting girls to avoid genetic conditions that affect only males (i.e., to avoid X-linked disease). Both trajectories emerged as a means to a medical rather than a lifestyle end. MicroSort and PGD arose and advanced in the animal reproductive sector, where clear industry interest drove the research. By the mid-1980s, both technologies were conceptually anticipated, and initial laboratory studies in nonhuman mammals proved by the end of that decade that they could successfully identify the sex of nonhuman embryos or sperm. Both were first experimentally demonstrated on rabbits and faced considerable technical obstacles in the move toward human application. This section traces the historical development of the technologies through two turns: from livestock industry to human therapeutic medicine and then on to human lifestyle medicine.

## Agriculture Industry—The Seedbed of Sex Selective ARTs

Just as the agricultural livestock industry provided the seedbed to all ARTs, so did it spur the development of sex selective ARTs (Clarke 1998). In the UK, PGD for humans was conceptually envisioned and publicly championed as a reproductive genetic technology, yet its first experimental demonstrations and clinical application were technically geared to select for sex. In fact, early references in the scientific literature refer to PGD as "embryo sexing" (Theodosiou and Johnson 2011, 458). "Sexing" refers to sex identification, a term used in scientific literature in relation to both embryos and sperm. PGD's first experimental demonstration came as early as 1968, when Robert Edwards, who received a Nobel Prize for advancing infertility medicine through the development of IVF, and Richard Gardner successfully biopsied cells from 119 rabbit embryos, sexed the embryos, and then transferred them back to rabbit does, which produced eighteen offspring all correctly sexed. Lawrence Johnson's first experimental demonstration of the Beltsville Sperm Sexing Technology (precursor to MicroSort), also on rabbits, occurred twenty-one years later, in 1989. The first clinical application in humans of the two technologies both occurred in the early 1990s.

Theodosiou and Johnson reason that the long time lag between the first experimental application in 1968 and the first human application of PGD in the 1990s was due to a lack of motivation to develop the method in humans. Although the early experimental development history of PGD is intertwined with that of IVF, IVF moved into the human clinical realm much earlier. Those in the UK involved with the advent of IVF, most famously Robert Edwards and Patrick Steptoe, never envisioned that IVF technology would only address infertility. In the experimental stages of IVF, long before the birth of Louise Brown, the first IVF baby, Edwards and Gardner, among others, simultaneously developed the technique of embryo biopsy used in PGD. As Edwards has emphasized in retrospective accounts of his work, PGD was *conceptualized* along with the possibility of fertilizing eggs outside of the womb (Edwards cited in Franklin and Roberts 2006, 42–43). Edwards, for example, applied for research funds to develop PGD in 1971, seven years before IVF was even successfully shown in humans. In the grant application Edwards proposed that a first potential application of PGD in humans could control "sex-linked mutant genes in man" (cited in Theodosiou and Johnson 2011, 461). Yet, the UK Medical Research Council rejected the proposal, and it was not until fifteen years later that UK scientists would form PROGRESS, a lobby to advocate for the realization of PGD that successfully drummed up public support. Thus, PGD development during the 1970s through the mid-1980s remained relegated to the animal agricultural sector.

The ability to control for sex in the production of farm animals, especially cattle, swine, and sheep, has long been recognized as having the ability to bring an economic boon to commercial agriculture (Johnson and Welch 1997, 337; Theodosiou and Johnson 2011, 459). This industry drove the development of both embryo and sperm sexing technologies during the 1970s and 1980s. David Karabinus, the scientific director of the US-based MicroSort human clinical trial (with a background in the field of animal reproduction), explains:

> Dr. Johnson [USDA scientist Lawrence Johnson, who developed the sperm-sexing technology branded "MicroSort" for humans] developed the application in livestock, because male cattle don't give milk, females do. Male cattle don't bear more young, females do. So, you don't need as many males as you do females to keep the line going to make babies. Female livestock are easier to manage. Males are more physical, bigger, and tend to be more aggressive. (IF 12/8/10–12/22/10)

In their history of the commercialization of sperm-sexing technologies within the cattle industry, Seidel and Garner (2008, 886–887) describe how dairy farmers would interpret the birth of several male cattle in a row as bad luck, resorting to "folkloric" (read: unscientific) ways to explain them. Dairy and meat farmers have long sought ways to reliably control the sex of their cattle, and the long-standing economic value of females in livestock reproduction spurred the development of both PGD and MicroSort. However, of the two technologies, MicroSort (or more accurately, its precursor, the Beltsville Sperm Sexing Technology) remains the preferred method within the industry because it can be applied with "artificial insemination."[1] PGD, on the other hand, requires IVF, a relatively complicated procedure that cannot easily be applied en masse. Optimizing sex selection for livestock reproduction must contend with industry standards that involve inseminating many cows at one time with the sperm of just one superior bull. Although PGD's design does not fit with that standard, the industry nonetheless remained interested in its development, in part because the experimental demonstration of sexing sperm took place much later (Theodosiou and Johnson 2011; personal communication with Larry Johnson, March 24, 2011).

During the 1970s and 1980s, then, research on PGD advanced within the realm of animal reproduction. PGD was demonstrated for sexing of sheep in 1975 and cattle in 1976. The timing of biopsy (stage of embryo development when cells are removed) and mode of analysis used to identify sex varied in these studies, none of which pointed to a potential application in humans (Theodosiou and Johnson 2011, 460). Similarly, the research that led to the development of MicroSort became technologically viable under the helm of the USDA, though the method was first conceptualized in a weapons laboratory through research funded by the US Department of Energy.

Scientists working at the Lawrence Livermore National Laboratory, a weapons lab in California, and the Max Planck Institute for Biochemistry in Munich, among other institutions, first theorized the potential of sperm sexing via flow cytometry (Van Dilla et al. 1977). Supported by the US Energy Research and Development Administration, this research studied the reproductive effects of radiation on humans (Van Dilla et al. 1977, Seidel and Garner 2008, Pinkel et al. 1982). The Livermore team described the purpose of the research thus: "The increasing presence of potentially hazardous substances in the environment makes it prudent to develop both tests for their genetic activity and methods to screen people for the effects of exposure. Reproductive effects are a major concern . . . *Because the presence of sperm with abnormal DNA content is a direct indication of genetic effects of exposure, we have explored the application of flow cytometric DNA content measurements to sperm*" (Pinkel et al. 1982, 1, emphasis mine). These scientists already knew of a relative DNA content difference between X- and Y-bearing sperm, and they anticipated that distinguishing between the two might be a by-product of their research. However, they certainly did not articulate a medical purpose for sexing human sperm, which did not appear in the literature until the early 1990s.

By the early 1980s, the Livermore scientists were able to detect relative DNA content differences between X and Y sperm populations based on fluorescence intensity after applying a DNA-binding fluorescing dye to tailless sperm. In 1982 they published their success in using flow cytometry to distinguish between X and Y sperm from bulls, rams, rabbits, and boars (Pinkel et al. 1982). Yet, these experiments did not yield live sorted sperm viable for reproduction, as the tails of the sperm had to be removed in order to get them to smoothly pass through the cytometer. The research on sexing sperm might have ended altogether had it not been subsequently taken up and funded by the USDA, prompted by a research proposal submitted by one of the Livermore scientists to the USDA while on sabbatical (Seidel and Garner 2008). While the Livermore lab had the advantage of being able to tinker with and improve various aspects of instrumentation (the USDA did not initially own a flow cytometer), the USDA had a clearer vested interest in pursuing research on sexing sperm. Lawrence Johnson, lead USDA scientist in the 1980s, recalls:

> So, I and Pinkel from Lawrence Livermore, which was a weapons laboratory, well, it still is, they had done some work with DNA and sperm, and they had demonstrated that if you stain the tailless sperm, the nuclei, what we call the heads, or whatever you want to call them, that you could demonstrate a DNA difference. And, so, but they had to get out of the business. They're Department of Energy, and they were looking initially at the effect of nuclear weapons on human sperm. So, that was the focus of their research when they got into the animals. (IF 9/14/10)

Thus, the Department of Energy would likely not have sustained ongoing research on sperm sorting for sexing purposes.

Several major technological developments in the 1980s shaped the practice. First, the standard cylindrical-shaped needle at the flow opening of the cytometer, which was better suited to the round shape of blood cells, was adapted to accommodate the flat-shaped heads of mammalian sperm (Pinkel et al. 1982, Johnson and Pinkel 1986).[2] Scientists had tried at first to imitate that round shape by removing the sperm tails, which meant the sperm could not be used in reproduction. Alongside tinkering with mechanical elements related to the cytometer design, which were ultimately incorporated into commercially available flow cytometers intended for use with sperm, scientists sought ways to change staining protocols because the dyes used in the early 1980s compromised the viability of the sperm (Johnson and Welch 1997, 345; Johnson et al. 1987). As Lawrence Johnson recalls,

> So, I said to Mary—actually, Mary Look, she was working for me at that time, this was about 1986—I said we need to just try it with in-tact sperm. I got ahead of myself. The stain we were using in the heads was detrimental to living sperm. So, I found another stain, and that's the Hoechst 33342 that's still used. It's the only one that works. (IF 9/14/10)

Once Dr. Johnson's team succeeded in getting viable sperm to flow through the cytometer, they separated X- from Y-bearing sperm populations and surgically inseminated that sperm in litter-bearing animals such as rabbits and pigs that rapidly produce a large number of offspring. The resulting proportions of sexed baby animals, they argued, could prove that the method worked. Figure 1.1 depicts Lawrence Johnson with a pig born using sorted sperm and IVF. In 1989, Dr. Johnson and two of his colleagues published the results of a rabbit study reporting that rabbit does inseminated with X-bearing sperm samples had a litter that was 94 percent female, and those inseminated with Y-bearing sperm had a litter that was 81 percent male (Johnson et al. 1989).

The paper "made waves," Johnson recalls. "It was a scientific breakthrough of considerable proportion because it had never been done before" (IF 9/14/10). As a postdoctoral student at South Dakota State University working in a flow cytometry lab, David Karabinus, who later

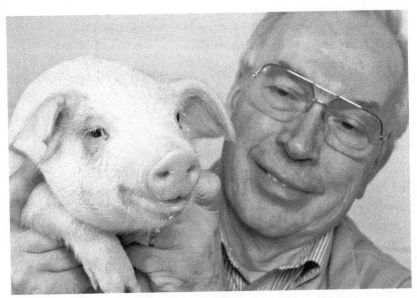

1.1. Dr. Johnson with sex preselected pig. Photograph by Keith Weller (K8409-9). Reprinted from *Agricultural Research Magazine* (Weaver-Missick 1999)

became the scientific director of the MicroSort human clinical trial, remembers when his advisor first brought Johnson's rabbit study to his attention: "To me that represented the epitome of science. It was a well thought out, well-based study, and the results were good, credible results. I just thought it was, as I told my postdoc advisor, I thought it was a landmark paper" (IF 12/8/10–10/22/10). The paper also caught the attention of scientists working in human genetics, especially Edward Fugger at the Genetics & IVF Institute (GIVF), whose background also stemmed from animal reproduction. Fugger, along with colleagues Joseph Schulman and Andrew Dorfman, took the initiative to approach Johnson about the prospects of applying the method in humans. Reaction to the paper thus ushered in a new collaboration between the USDA and GIVF that would lead to the transfer of the method to human medicine. Scientific collaboration of concern in the history of MicroSort shifted from Livermore and the USDA to the USDA and GIVF. The purpose of the research shifted along with these institutional changes. By the end of the 1980s, both PGD and MicroSort's antecedent in agriculture had been successfully shown to sex nonhuman mammals, and both technologies were poised to enter human medicine.

## "A powerful approach to disease prevention"— The Transfer to Human Medicine

When PGD researchers began to direct their efforts toward application in humans after 1986–1987, the stated reason was medical: to avoid X-linked genetic disease with an eventual expansion to screen against other genetic conditions. UK scientists sought to *publicly* safeguard the practice of IVF by fostering a political climate supportive of their research on human applications of PGD against a growing threat from anti-abortion interests. The scientists' advocacy imbued the technology with a social validity and paved the way for *disassociation* from abortion, which lifestyle sex selection has further advanced.

In Britain, the emergence of PGD coincided with the establishment of the UK's (and the world's) first state authority to regulate embryo research and the practice of assisted reproductive medicine. In their ethnographic study of PGD, Sarah Franklin and Celia Roberts trace a critical period (1984–1991) in the intertwined histories of the technology and the national regulatory body. The authors draw attention to the "role of PGD in focusing and clarifying public attitudes toward reproductive biomedicine" during that period, stressing PGD's very public form due to a multiplicity of representations in media and in parliamentary debates (2006, 92, 39). Theodosiou and Johnson, in their historical study of the motivations to achieve PGD, also pinpoint 1986–1987 as the year "pivotal" to "clinically oriented PGD interest," driven in part by changing attitudes toward prenatal diagnostic technologies (PND) and IVF, but also significantly "stimulated" by a charged political climate in which embryo research came under attack by an anti-abortion bloc of parliamentarians (2011, 467). Both studies highlight how technological development takes place not only in the lab but also in the social and political sphere.

Scientists were motivated to develop PGD in part as a means of demonstrating the medical importance of embryo research beyond the treatment of infertility. Within the situated context of mid-1980s Britain, proposed anti-abortion legislation began to widen its ambit from debates about shortening the timing of legal abortion during pregnancy to banning embryo research and IVF practice. Alarmed by what was at stake, UK scientists and clinicians organized to defend a publicly made case to support the clinical practice of IVF as well as the development of IVF-dependent technologies, including PGD. They recommended that research be publicly financed and proceed within the bounds of a responsible governing authority (what became Britain's highly acclaimed Human Fertilisation and Embryology Authority [HFEA]), which would ensure their "proper" use. Scientists and clinicians took pains to associate PGD foremost with its medical indication (i.e., its application in the realm of clinical genetics as a preventive/therapeutic intervention), and to disassociate it from controversial and commercial uses, including improving IVF success rates, much less being used as a means of lifestyle sex selection. In their historical account of PGD, Franklin and Roberts explain,

> Britain's place in the wider global context of PGD can . . . be described as medically and scientifically progressive, but cautious in relation to uses of PGD that could be seen as too commercial—including the "boutique" choice of sex preselection and the high-priced niche market in aneuploidy detection [i.e., checking chromosome numbers as a means of reducing IVF failure]. Although Britain is not the largest provider of PGD in global terms, its scientific contributions to the technique have continued to be distinguished since PGD's first successful implementation in London in 1990. This is in part because the medical-scientific community in Britain has sought to protect the image of PGD by minimizing its association with fertility enhancement and emphasizing its "original" role as a branch of clinical genetics. (2006, 98–99)

As Britain's scientists defined "proper" uses of PGD as a means of "minimizing public 'discomfort'" with the new technology, it also, in making the medical argument for PGD, highlighted the technology's ability to obviate abortion in reproductive genetics. Scientists pursued the development of PGD publicly and in active, direct response to anti-abortion legislation threatening embryo research, emphasizing the technology's ability to avoid repeat and late-term abortions associated with a positive amniocentesis result.

Within mid-1980s Britain, then, the normalization of prenatal diagnostic technologies (PND) and IVF, on the one hand, and the encroachment of anti-abortion forces on embryology and IVF practice on the other, formed the contextual backdrop to public debates in which scientists articulated a need to pursue the development of PGD. In June 1985, an anti-abortion bill put forth by conservative MP Enoch Powell would have ended research on embryos in Britain if not for a narrow defeat. Members of PROGRESS began to persuasively advocate for PGD as urgently needed by inheritable genetic disease patients, who had to contend with the "fear and anxiety" associated with pregnancies terminated after positive PND results. In a 1987 assessment of prospects for PGD, McLaren and Penketh highlighted not the relative simplicity of PND vis-à-vis PGD, as McLaren had done just two years earlier, but PND's associated "high physical and emotional price," necessitating tentative pregnancies and possible repeat abortions (Penketh and McLaren 1987, 747, cited in Franklin and Roberts 2006, 56; Rothman 1993). The UK parliamentary debate on timing of abortion and research on embryos thus helped to spur the first articulations of a medically justifiable need for PGD—a clearly spelled out *medical* problem (early childhood death and disease affliction) requiring a *medical* solution. As it turned out, this motivation not only served the development of PGD by instigating an increased pace in research, but also set the stage for MicroSort's entrée into human medicine just a few years later.

Initial technical obstacles facing PGD research for humans resolved over time through the concurrent development of requisite in vitro technologies such as IVF and PCR (polymerase chain reaction). IVF produced the raw material—human embryos—and PCR provided the initial diagnostic means to identify sex because it could quickly amplify (or reproduce) DNA, thus requiring the removal of only a single cell from the embryos. The first clinical application of PGD took place in 1990 by Alan Handyside and Robert Winston. Using PCR to amplify Y-chromosome-specific DNA strands, the clinicians isolated female embryos for transfer. Once again, sex selection took place in this initial clinical instantiation as a means of avoiding the birth of male children; females can carry but do not express the disease trait.

Although the first human application of PGD provided the *explicit* scientific proof that PGD could be useful in clinical genetics, it *implicitly* and simultaneously proved itself as a viable new human sexing technology. UK scientists Penketh and McLaren made their points in support of PGD development with specific reference to beta-thalassemia, which is not a sex-linked disease, but much of the experimental research studies into PGD taking place between 1986 and 1990 (a period of vibrant and fast-paced experimentation in the UK) focused on attempts to sex embryos in order to avoid sex-linked genetic disease (Franklin and Roberts 2006, 52; Theodosiou and Johnson 2011, 462). The majority of sex-linked diseases (examples are hemophilia and Duchenne muscular dystrophy) are X-linked, meaning that the disease only expresses itself in male children, so selecting for a girl avoids the 25 percent chance of having an affected child. Used in this way, PGD does not actually screen for the genetic mutation itself; rather, it screens for the presence of the Y chromosome. In effect, the process involves sex selection. I make this point not to question sex selective PGD as a tool of genetic medicine, but to highlight that, in material-technological terms, that first human clinical instantiation of PGD in 1990 demonstrated the technology as viable for human sex selection in general, including but also beyond its medically therapeutic intent. The combination of wider genetic screening potential and actual technical ability to sex embryos made PGD a potent tool for lifestyle sex selection, one that at once supplied a medical justification for pursuing it and also an effective material-technical capability to screen for sex.

Today, the method of using sex selective PGD to screen against sex-linked diseases appears somewhat crude, as advances in the technology allow PGD to identify more of the specific disease mutations in DNA that happen to also be sex-linked. In this way PGD use can actually prevent the implantation of any embryo, male or female, that is either afflicted with or a carrier of the disease (Sermon et al. 2004, Ogilvie et al. 2005). Scientists anticipated a decline in medically indicated sex selective PGD use by the early 2000s. In fact, in 2002 the PGD Consortium of the European Society of Human Reproduction and Embryology reported a drop in the number of PGD cases involving sexing to avoid X-linked disease (ESHRE PGD Consortium Steering Committee 2002, 243–244).

The scope of PGD applications has broadened considerably since the first clinical use of this technology. Although PCR was initially used for embryo sex identification, in practice FISH soon replaced PCR as the "diagnostic" technique of choice because it provided a simpler means to test for chromosomal sex and numbers (Sermon et al. 2004, 1633). A method for detecting and mapping sequences of genes within chromosomes that came into being during the 1980s, FISH was among a number of new techniques that revolutionized the field of molecular genetics, providing an important diagnostic tool to check for chromosomal abnormalities and genetic mutations (Levsky and Singer 2003). FISH was already well integrated as a PND tool of analysis when its utility for PGD and MicroSort was first realized. While the utility of FISH allowed PGD sex and aneuploidy screening to become more widespread and accessible, the method, it turns out, also provided a critical key to the overall development of MicroSort. GIVF scientists who pursued an application of the Beltsville Sperm Sexing Technology in humans told Johnson that they were interested in the method's potential to avoid sex-linked genetic disease in human babies (IF 9/14/10). Johnson anticipated initial technical challenges. First, relative to sperm in other mammals, human X- and Y-bearing sperm have a small difference in DNA content (see figure 1.2). Initial experiments to sort X- from Y-bearing sperm were conducted on mammals with larger differences in the DNA content of their sex chromosomes, such as the vole (9 percent) or chinchilla (7.5 percent) as compared to the bull (3.8 percent) or the human (2.8 percent).

Moreover, this smaller difference in DNA content between human sex chromosomes compromised the utility of Johnson's own method of determining sort purity (through a reanalysis of the sorted sperm populations, which involved putting them again through the flow cytometer). The GIVF team had a solution to offer: FISH.

Founded by Joseph Schulman in 1984, GIVF uniquely provided under one institutional roof an IVF clinical facility, a molecular genetics lab that provided prenatal diagnostic services to pregnant women, and one of the largest sperm banks in the US. FISH was one technique already in use in GIVF's genetic laboratory as a means to analyze fetal and placental tissues, and according to GIVF's website, Shulman realized its potential to serve as a reliable test of purity of the sorted sperm samples. Furthermore, GIVF, through its sperm cryobank, could readily supply the raw material needed for the experiments. While the USDA now had the flow cytometer and the expertise with the instrumentation needed to make adaptations for human sperm, GIVF supplied the human sperm itself and the test needed to check the proportions of X or Y sperm populations. The proximity of the two institutions (about twenty-five miles

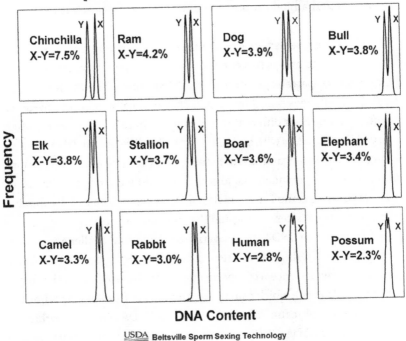

# Sperm Sort Separations

Frequency

| | | | |
|---|---|---|---|
| **Chinchilla** X-Y=7.5% | **Ram** X-Y=4.2% | **Dog** X-Y=3.9% | **Bull** X-Y=3.8% |
| **Elk** X-Y=3.8% | **Stallion** X-Y=3.7% | **Boar** X-Y=3.6% | **Elephant** X-Y=3.4% |
| **Camel** X-Y=3.3% | **Rabbit** X-Y=3.0% | **Human** X-Y=2.8% | **Possum** X-Y=2.3% |

DNA Content

USDA Beltsville Sperm Sexing Technology

1.2. Difference in DNA content between X- and Y-bearing sperm in different animal species. I thank H. David Guthrie of the USDA for the use of this figure from his presentation "Animal Biosciences and Biotechnology Laboratory 'Gender Pre-selection'" (n.d.).

distance between Fairfax, VA, and Beltsville, MD) likely simplified the effort.[3] Since the research was mainly conducted at the USDA lab, a USDA restriction that prohibited using the sperm for fertilization of human eggs effectively limited the study to determining only whether the Beltsville technology could reliably distinguish and separate X from Y viable human sperm.

In 1993 the USDA-GIVF collaboration published their findings. The article proposes the development of human sperm sexing as "a powerful approach to disease prevention" (Johnson et al. 1993, 1733) that "could in time reduce or eliminate the use of selective abortion as a means of decreasing the incidence of X-linked genetic disorders" (1738). The authors make no mention of sex selection as a lifestyle option, highlighting instead a medical purpose and a disassociation with selective abortion.

FISH results revealed enriched samples of X and Y sperm populations with an average 82 and 75 percent rate of purity, respectively, as opposed to their normal 50 percent presence in unsorted semen. Yet, the results also stress the challenges posed by human sperm in comparison to livestock sperm, including their different morphology—more angular heads (rather than paddle-shaped, as with bull sperm), smaller difference in DNA content, as already mentioned, and sperm heterogeneity (lack of uniformity among sperm from a single individual and between individuals) (Johnson et al. 1993, 1735). These complicating material factors compromised the number of sperm retrieved after sorting and the sort sample purities.

For some at the USDA, the material-technological challenges of morphology and DNA difference seemed daunting. By 1993 the USDA had gained ample experience with sperm sorting for livestock varieties (especially bull and swine), which could potentially move from the experimental to the commercial realm. Yet Glenn Welch, a USDA scientist working in the 1990s in the USDA-GIVF collaboration, recalls having a "negative attitude" to the prospects for commercialization of the Beltsville Sperm Sexing Technology. Welch thought the method was too expensive and labor intensive to work well in the cattle industry, and the relatively smaller difference between X and Y DNA content in human sperm meant there would always be a greater amount of overlap in X and Y subpopulations compromising sort purity.

Welch explained to me why MicroSort typically produces purer X sorts, biasing the technology toward a more effective production of females. The process relies on measuring the relative strength of fluorescence of a dye that binds to DNA, and since Y sperm have less DNA than X sperm, they fluoresce less. Y sperm are unlikely to overfluoresce and fall into the X tube; however, issues with stain process impacted by the "quality" of the sperm might allow an X sperm to fluoresce less than it otherwise could, and therefore be read falsely by the cytometer as a Y. Bovine sperm sorting, on the other hand, has been reported to produce far less disparity in sort purity between X and Y samples, with both ranging from 90 to 95 percent (FN 9/10/10, Gosálvez et al. 2011).

In addition to the disparity in average rates of purity between X and Y human sperm samples, purity rates vary between individuals. Fugger et al. point out the challenge of heterogeneity both within the sperm of one individual and between individuals (1998, 2369). Although Lawrence Johnson and Glenn Welch of the USDA asserted in 1997 that it would be "essential" to "prevalidate" sort purity *before* using sorted sperm with ARTs in human reproduction, in clinical use this has proved logistically difficult. Due to the additional time necessary to conduct purity tests, clinicians and their patients who wish to utilize fresh samples directly after sorting will not know the results of the purity of their individual sample.[4] The scientific director explained that the 88 percent average purity rate for an X-sort noted on MicroSort informational materials is sometimes misinterpreted as guaranteed:

> We've had an X-sort as high as 99 percent, and we've had X-sorts down in the 60 percent range. That's one of the things that patients don't think about. It's an average, and an average is just that. It's the high ones and the low ones added together and divided by the number of sorts. It gives you an average, so you have a range. (IF 12/8/10–12/22/10)

Human sperm heterogeneity within one individual sample also posed a challenge for developers of MicroSort. Reproductive scientists interpret such heterogeneity, which they say results from a lack of selective breeding, as a marker of poor sperm "quality." The scientific director of the MicroSort clinical trial explained:

> So in the livestock species males and females both have been selected for reproductive performance, and on the male side, a big factor in reproductive performance is not only sperm numbers but sperm quality. By and large bulls, boars, rams, produce sperm that look like they've been cut out of cookie cutters—very, very uniform. Humans have not been selected for reproductive performance. Compared to bull sperm, humans produce really, really crappy sperm. (IF 12/8/10–12/22/10)

Lawrence Johnson, inventor of the technology, made a similar comparison while explaining the impact of human sperm heterogeneity:

Interesting in animals there's been a lot more selection because the use of livestock obviously for procreating, improvement, and this sort of thing, whereas the human population that is not the case. Human sperm, their DNA is quite, if you can visualize a sperm head, and there are pockets that are less dense with DNA. They call it vacuoles a lot of times. So, you have a lot more of them in the human sperm. In livestock sperm you have very little of that. They're very uniform. And part of the staining process is uniformity of the stain to get your stain into the sperm uniformly at a level where you have a minimum of variable. (IF 9/14/10)

The heterogenic form of human sperm—lack of uniformity as a result of a lack of selective breeding—actually forms a kind of material resistance to the process in general.

In spite of Welch's doubts, the commercialization of bovine sperm sorting proceeded with the establishment of multiple sorter sites (eighteen for just one company called Sexing Technologies), each outfitted with multiple flow cytometers. Some individual sorting sites even have ten flow cytometers running side by side for fourteen hours a day (IF 9/14/10, Sexing Technologies LLC 2012). This scale does not translate to human reproduction due to both the material characteristics of human sperm and the social and cultural practices of human reproduction, which disallow the insemination of many women with just one man's sperm. Indeed, the transition from livestock to human reproduction required *material* as well as *institutional* translation. Waldby and Cooper describe a similar translation with respect to IVF: "The technology of human IVF emerged from the livestock industry although in institutional and economic terms it was never organized along the same lines of mass reproduction that reigned in the livestock industry. Human reproductive IVF does not involve reordering the developmental biology of cells . . . . The process is organized precisely to *preserve* the ontogenic and teleological potentials of the germinal cells" (Waldby and Cooper 2010, 15). Relative to livestock reproduction, then, the social and cultural practices of human reproduction, combined with the material conditions of human sperm morphology, heterogeneity, and lower DNA difference between human X and Y sperm, impacted the sex-sorting process in a way that defied mass use and did not as effectively produce boys. While the precursor to MicroSort (the

Beltsville Sperm Sexing Technology) has the design potential to be applied en masse through artificial insemination, its human application does not. In the meaning-making shift to human medicine, however, such material impediments dissolve, as the purpose of the technology shifts from mass production of female livestock to reducing the likelihood of X-linked disease expression in human babies.

Although the GIVF-USDA collaboration proved that the method could work in theory, in practice the safety and efficacy of the method ultimately to produce human babies of desired sex still had to be shown. *Institutionally*, the locus of research had to shift once more. In 1992, GIVF took over the task. The Office of Technology Transfer of the Agricultural Research Services of the USDA granted GIVF a seventeen-year exclusive license to develop the Beltsville Sperm Sexing Technology for commercial use in humans. Johnson claims to have had at least in one aspect significant influence on that process:

> One impact that I did have early on was the technology transfer. They wanted to put one license across the board, animals and humans, and not have any distinction. Absolutely not in my view. And they did take my advice at that time to separate them, so that you have a separate license for humans. Because you got different people dealing with it. You've got people trained in medicine, human medicine, that need to be working with humans. That's indeed where their clientele is. Whereas the whole animal world is a whole different set of circumstances. (IF 9/14/10)

In this way, this history of sperm sexing divided, with a boundary between human and nonhuman development sharply drawn. GIVF purchased two flow cytometers, secured institutional review board (IRB) approval from Inova Fairfax Hospital (Wadman 2001), and in 1993 the human clinical trial was under way. GIVF named the human application "MicroSort."

## Medicalization and the Anticipation of Lifestyle Applications

In a 1995 report of the first achieved MicroSort pregnancy published in the scientific journal *Human Reproduction*, trial scientists proposed a material linkage between MicroSort and PGD in which MicroSort would serve as an "adjunct" to PGD "for the prevention of X-linked disease" (Levinson et al. 1995, 979). The combination, the authors contended, raised the chance of pregnancy by increasing the number of female embryos (as identified by PGD) from which to choose for transfer. Further, they suggested that MicroSort combined with PGD would simultaneously minimize the number of male embryos, the production of which posed a "dilemma" for patients as some might be unaffected by disease (979).[5] In fact, the first human clinical instantiations of MicroSort did the reverse by utilizing PGD as an adjunct of sorts, a backup and further test of validation—"purely a necessary precaution to check the sex ratio and to identify the rare male embryos conceived by the few Y spermatozoa which escaped X-sorting" (Edwards and Beard 2005, 978). In this way, at the very moment MicroSort was introduced to scientists in the field as a viable, sex selective technology in human reproduction, the parallel histories of MicroSort and PGD converged within the framework of scientific discussions of sexing for medical purposes.

An editorial introducing the paper, coauthored by reproductive scientists Robert Edwards and Helen K. Beard, reinforced that frame while also anticipating the leap to lifestyle sex selection. Entitled "Sexing Human Spermatozoa to Control Sex Ratios at Birth Is Now a Reality," the editorial first granted MicroSort a high level of scientific recognition—another form of validation—coming from some of Europe's most esteemed scientists in the field. This editorial support granted to MicroSort's first pregnancy may in no small part have been influenced by the enduring friendship and growing affinity between GIVF's Schulman and Robert Edwards, which first began while Schulman attended Cambridge in the mid-1970s, where he had the opportunity to observe early (unsuccessful) attempts to clinically apply IVF (Schulman 2010). Second, the editorial seals the material convergence of MicroSort and PGD as sexing technology alternatives (if not adjuncts) by discussing the two in relation to each other. The authors wrote:

> Sperm sorting will be a valuable adjunct to other forms of very early prenatal diagnosis. It could well replace the use of preimplantation diagnosis which utilizes marker genes on the X and Y chromosomes

for sexing. Preimplantation diagnosis offers a high degree of success, perhaps equal to or greater than sperm sorting, but it is an expensive approach to diagnosis. Its great advantage is avoiding or reducing the need for abortion, but it involves an operation on the wife, IVF, and the rejection of the afflicted embryos. (Edwards and Beard 1995, 977–978)

Here, as in subsequent comparative assessments of the technologies, the authors not only presume heteronormative applications of both technologies, but also that MicroSort will most likely be combined with insemination procedures (unlike PGD, which necessitates IVF). Finally and most significantly, Edwards and Beard foreshadow the immediately forthcoming move made by MicroSort to expand to nonmedical uses. They condition the acceptability of using MicroSort for "sex choice" with its inherent capability (unlike PGD) to be combined with "artificial insemination." They stated, "The introduction of sex choice *using artificial insemination* with sorted spermatozoa would make the method highly acceptable for sexing for social purposes. Indeed, such an approach may be imminent" (978, emphasis mine). In fact, the USDA license that extended MicoSort indications to what today is described as *family balancing* was deliberated and approved that very year. Edwards and Beard continued, "This prospect will rattle the skeletons in the cupboard for some observers as they contemplate the ethics of a further example of a rapidly advancing biotechnology" (978). The anticipated move to lifestyle sex selection found even earlier expression in an opinion piece published in 1993 by GIVF founder Joseph D. Schulman.

Thus, at the moment of its very introduction into human medicine, even as MicroSort's *medical* purpose was still being mobilized and the technology's viability for human applications was undergoing its earliest testing, developers not only envisioned future human lifestyle applications but also began to disassociate both MicroSort and PGD from abortion technologies. Schulman's piece foreshadows the "family balancing" policy later operationalized within GIVF.

The *initial* applications of human sperm sorting are likely to be limited, and to achieve broad ethical acceptance. . . . It will be applied prior to medical fertilization in families at high risk of bearing children with serious X-linked diseases . . . In this application, the sorting would achieve the laudable goals of reducing the incidence of X-linked diseases *and decreasing the frequency of pregnancy terminations after prenatal diagnosis.* The only available alternative for achieving both of these goals, IVF with preimplantation genetic testing, is complex, difficult, expensive, and necessitates the destruction of embryos.

What carefully defined conditions would permit more ethically acceptable gender preselection of healthy girls or boys? The "balancing" of sex ratios in families is certain to attract considerable discussion in this regard. Consider a family with its only children being three healthy boys. If a fourth child is desired, and a girl is preferred by the parents, why would sperm sorting to enhance the odds of a female not be ethical?

In my opinion, many people will conclude that ethically acceptable guidelines for family balancing can and should be developed. One position to be considered might simply be that it is ethical to perform balancing to increase the less represented gender in any family that already has at least one child. (Schulman 1993, 1541, emphasis mine)

Schulman's assertion of a medical need for MicroSort simultaneously looks ahead to the potential for lifestyle uses, long before such applications would also envelope PGD. His language asserting a lifestyle iteration of sex selection within ART is enabled by material aspects of MicroSort's design, for example, its bias toward the more effective production of girls (Schulman's hypothetical family of three boys would likely not have been randomly chosen), and its relative simplicity and lower risk profile than PGD (assumed as it was to be applied with IUI instead of IVF). Attributing the idea to Schulman and Edwards and Beard, bioethicist Guido Pennings in Belgium wrote an extended argument to defend family balancing "as a morally acceptable application of sex selection" when restricted to serving couples with at least one child and selecting for the less represented sex (1996, 2339). Family balancing thereby began its moves from a speculative idea to a full-blown discourse.

To summarize the parallels, PGD and MicroSort developed on distinct pathways with significant technical obstacles to overcome during the 1970s and 1980s in the research realm of animal agriculture, where each technology was prized for its capability to produce female livestock. The potential for human applications could not sustain the development of these technologies initially, and in their eventual transfer to human medicine, both technologies underwent a process of redefinition, transforming from the goal of female livestock selection to a means of avoiding sex-linked disease in humans. Therefore, the emergence of the technologies alone could not preclude or determine the construction of lifestyle sex selection.

Initial human trials demonstrated foremost in material terms their viability as sexing technologies, even when this function was applied as a means to the end of avoiding disease. These development pathways converged materially as scientists framed the arrival of MicroSort in connection to PGD, as an adjunct or alternative technology within the larger clinical worlds of fertility and reproductive genetic medicine. The coincident timing of arrival of MicroSort and PGD paved the way for their combination into a new set of "high-tech" human sex selection practices. Their first convergence took place within highly integrated scientific and clinical spheres of molecular genetics and reproductive medicine, in which information and technologies fused toward their *medicalization*, with PGD leading the way. This process served as a stepping stone to their subsequent *biomedicalization*, as they became a set of alternative technoscientific interventions designed to fulfill, as first asserted by MicroSort, consumer lifestyle desires.

## Situating Lifestyle Sex Selection

In the *Global Biopolitics of the IUD*, Chikako Takeshita writes a "biography of an artifact" exploring how IUD devices embody what she calls biopolitical scripts that "involve three way co-configurations of technologies, users, and modes of governance over the body" (Takeshita 2012, 4, 28). Combining STS approaches with intersectionality and Foucauldian theories of biopower, she explores how these scripts produce meanings that stratify IUDs-users-bodies in the United States and globally. For example, Takeshita contrasts the "next generation," life-enhancing, contemporary user of a menses-suppressing Mirena IUD with the "less modern," overfertile user of the cheaper ParaGard IUD in the non-West (140, 149). In a similar way, I crudely trace here the identities of MicroSort and PGD as they accrue meanings in relation or in contrast to other technologies in a way that can mark differences among users.

# Home within Fertility Inc.—Technologies of Association

Situated within the overlapping Western worlds of high-tech reproductive medicine and clinical genetics, the tools of lifestyle sex selection get charged by the "promissory capital" and "hope and hype" of fast-paced change in biotechnology (Thompson 2005; Adams et al. 2009, 252). Both PGD and MicroSort preclude the simplest method—vaginal insemination that can be applied by a user at home—since PGD requires IVF, and the application of MicroSort decreases sperm numbers to an extent that renders vaginal insemination ineffective. An intrauterine (as opposed to vaginal) insemination can improve the chance of establishing a pregnancy when sperm numbers are low, but IUI requires professional assistance in most cases since the catheter that releases the sperm must breach a woman's cervix. In the hands of ART providers and within the walls of Fertility Inc., both MicroSort and PGD have been swept up in processes that normalize, routinize, and "ratchet up" technological interventions in order to optimize the chance of pregnancy (Thompson 2005; Mamo 2007, 165).

By the time MicroSort and PGD entered human medicine in the 1990s, IVF had moved from a highly controversial technology to one that was beginning to normalize. IVF has material-technological significance because it produces the embryos, the "raw material" required to conduct PGD. Moreover, the context of IVF normalization provided lifestyle sex selection technologies with an associative "home" in fertility clinics. Cussins's ethnographic account of practices in US fertility clinics describes the techniques by which the strangeness and novelty of IVF practice became "natural," "normal," and "routine" (Cussins 1998, 67). Indeed, as Franklin and Roberts argue, the push for PGD in the UK, in which IVF functioned as a requisite technology, "helped to establish its [IVF's] social and political legitimacy" (Franklin and Roberts 2006, 60). As IVF proceeded to normalize, its meanings as a tool for family building and pregnancy making (rather than terminating), as well as a "hope technology," deepened its associations with valued reproduction (Franklin 1997). MicroSort and PGD latch onto these sites of meaning.

Emerging in the 1990s, intracytoplasmic sperm injection (ICSI) is an IVF process to fertilize eggs that physically micro-injects a single sperm into an egg rather than relying on spontaneous fertilization after placing eggs and sperm together in a petri dish, as in traditional IVF. Traditional IVF sometimes results in some eggs remaining unfertilized. Originally, reproductive scientists developed ICSI to address male factor infertility marked by low sperm count or impaired sperm motility or morphology (Sherins et al. 1995). Yet, at two US clinics I visited, ICSI is today routinely applied with IVF to ensure that all available eggs become fertilized. All providers I spoke to in the field confirmed this trend both inside and outside the US. Routine use of ICSI with IVF has the potential to erase both the medically defined problem of male infertility (for which it has served as a medical treatment) and the concomitant sociocultural negotiations (see Inhorn 2012 on Arab masculinities). For MicroSort, which induces low sperm counts especially when combined with sperm freezing, ICSI is a highly significant addition to sex selective ART. Discussing the compounding stresses that sperm undergo through freeze-thaw cycles in conjunction with MicroSort, the scientific director of the trial pointed out the compensatory function of ICSI: "The good news is for an ICSI cycle, you don't need really vigorously motile sperm, because they're going to inject the sperm anyway. All they need to be is twitching" (12/8/10–12/22/10). Thus, in the quest for IVF success that involves a ratcheting up of technologies, today's routine use of ICSI (with IVF) counteracts compromised reproductive viability in sperm as induced by MicroSort combined with freeze-thaw processes.

## Technologies of Disassociation

Situated within the dominant position of "modern Western sciences" (Harding 2006, 1), developers of MicroSort and PGD disassociated these techniques from other kinds of sex selection practices. The assertion of scientific validity in relation to preexisting preconception methods such as Shettles or Ericsson helped to justify a medical application of MicroSort. Scientists asserted that MicroSort and PGD *really* work, unlike "pseudoscientific" or unscientific methods that falsely make the claim to sway the odds of getting a boy or girl. Further, they distanced sex selective ART from the politically illegitimate category of sex selective abortion.

## "Pseudoscientific" Preconception Interventions

The website mygenderselection.com, for example, contrasts MicroSort and PGD with the "pseudoscience" of Shettles and Ericsson, both preconception methods of sex selection that became popular in the 1970s (http://mygenderselection.com/the-pseudoscience, accessed March 16, 2012). MicroSort, in particular, had the added charge of demonstrating scientific validity in the face of similar methods whose legitimacy had come under question. Named after their founders, Landrum B. Shettles and Ronald Ericsson, both methods claimed to be scientific because their basis of action relied on codified knowledge existing since the early twentieth century that it is the sex chromosome of the sperm that contributes to human sex differentiation.[6] Both Shettles and Ericsson theorized that Y sperm swim faster than X sperm, basing their methods of intervention on this difference. Competing scientists dismissed the claims made by Shettles and Ericsson since the Shettles method did not pass the basic scientific principle of repeatability, and the sought-after enriched X- or Y-bearing populations of sperm produced via the Ericsson method could not be independently verified on a consistent basis (Claassens et al. 1995, Flaherty et al. 1997, Rose and Wong 1998, Fugger et al. 1998).

The motivation to undo the potential harm of pre-conception methods that made false claims partially propelled the research for a viable, scientifically based method of sperm sexing forward. USDA scientist Lawrence Johnson described to me his own contention with what he called "shysters," those "who were in the field to try to make a buck, with little concern for scientific merit or for the farmers they swindled. I probably analyzed five hundred samples from forty or so similar 'shysters' with 50:50 results [i.e., after sorting, the proportions of X and Y sperm were still 50:50]" (personal communication, March 11, 2011). In one of their few articles written on the application of the Beltsville Sperm Sexing Technology in humans, Lawrence Johnson and Glenn Welch cite studies that discredit the Ericsson method and present their own method as one that "enhances the credibility" though it does not "still the controversy" surrounding its use in humans (1997, 338). As Johnson asserts, "Anyone can run a sperm through a cell sorter, but if you cannot verify what you have done, it has no merit" (personal communication, March 11, 2011). In his description of how he became a provider of MicroSort and PGD, one clinic director told me that it was precisely his concern that patients were given false information about the potential of an Ericsson-like method he observed in use that prompted him to look into newer methods.[7]

> We were also starting to do PGD at that point, and so on several patients that were doing PGD they had these gradient heightened procedures done on the sperm (a method similar to Ericsson), and then we looked at the outcome to see what the gender of the embryos were, and it was 50:50, you know. So, it didn't do anything. And, we also did internal examinations where we did FISH on sperm that was either prepared in our gender selection method or just the way we always do it, and found no difference in the ratios, so at that point, I stopped doing it, and I got in touch with MicroSort . . . I'm a patient advocate, and that's what led me to look into gender selection in the first place, because I thought we were potentially providing people with false hope, and I don't like to do that. (IF 9/9/10)

Thus, researchers and later providers had a stake in maintaining a sharp boundary between their own and other preconception methods they deemed "unscientific." In this way, they could harness recognition, legitimacy, and other types of value associated with high science.

## Scientific Methods Involving Abortion

Other relevant battles for legitimacy in this story were waged a half-century earlier. In *Disciplining Reproduction*, Adele Clarke documents the historical processes of negotiation between reproductive scientists and birth control advocates (of various stripes) during the first half of the twentieth century to pursue research on contraception. Among their demands, a "redirection of contraceptive research" toward more complex and systemic approaches began the process of turning contraceptives into "scientific solutions" (Clarke 1998, 263, 192). In general, Clarke describes the struggles by the reproductive sciences to overcome several forces of illegitimacy (237–248), from associations with sexuality to "controversial social movements" (241) to "clinical quackery" (242). For some of these same overlapping reasons, the medical profession did not rush to claim jurisdiction over abortion. On the contrary, as several scholars have documented, the professionalization of US medicine in the late nineteenth century occurred in part through campaigning by the newly formed American Medical Association to criminalize abortion (Riessman 1983, Halfmann 2011). Even after legalization in the US in 1973, the medical establishment did not fully embrace abortion as being in its domain in part because most abortions occur in freestanding clinics apart from "mainstream" practices, and providers are sometimes still viewed within the profession as "low skilled 'profiteer(s)'" (Halfmann 2011, 201). As sociologist Drew Halfmann asserts, medicalization is a "continuous value," or a process, rather than a "category or state" (186). As such, it occurs relative to other processes. His historical case study of abortion in the US describes how medicalization and demedicalization often occurred simultaneously. His typology assists in discerning the ways in which disassociation (or gatekeeping) can at once fortify the biomedicalization of sex selective ART and also reinforce the nonmedicalization of other practices, such as sex selective abortion.

Population control advocates backed by philanthropy prompted the incorporation of birth control within the reproductive sciences, but an attempt to do the same for sex selective abortion did not succeed. In her history of the connections between the implementation of population control strategies and the rise of sex selective abortion in India, Mara Hvistendahl documents that beginning in 1975, sex detection by amniocentesis followed by sex selective abortions was introduced in Indian government hospitals as a means of reducing population growth (2011, 81). Papers delivered at an Indian national conference of pediatricians at the time promoted the method as a form of family planning (82). Studies from as far back as the 1950s by population scientists in international arenas identified son preference as a significant factor influencing fertility in India (86). The intense globally applied political pressure to assert population control in developing countries in the 1970s led to some of the most egregious violations of reproductive rights in history, including the sterilization of 6.2 million men in India during the late 1970s period of antidemocratic, authoritarian "emergency" rule (88).

According to Hvistendahl, it was precisely within this mid-1970s context of pressure to control population growth that the medical director of the Population Council, Sheldon Segal, played a role in the development of an amniocentesis trial at the All-India Institute of Medical Sciences to detect and abort female fetuses for the sake of reducing fertility (85–86). However, responding to protests by Indian feminists and allied groups, India's health minister stopped the trial within government hospitals, but the method continued to proliferate in private clinics (82). In the mid-1980s, primarily advertisements by private clinics and physician anecdotes, rather than sex ratios, propelled activists into action again. For the most part, a link—let alone a definitive causal link between sex selective abortion and declining sex ratios—did not feature in the earliest years of the campaign against sex selection in India (Mazumdar 2003, FASDSP 2003, Gupte 2003). The discursive turn to connect sex selection with population sex ratio imbalance began after the 1991 census, and as part of a strategic plan to appeal to the central government for regulatory action on the issue (Ravindra 1993). The possibility of this convergence arose because of parallel scholarly and activist attention on the sex ratio. Spurred by broadening social movement protests, the Government of India passed the Prenatal Diagnostic Techniques Act in 1994 to outlaw the use of PND for nonmedical sex determination. This occurred in tandem with the first internationally articulated condemnation of sex selective abortions that same year at the International Conference on Population and Development in Cairo. Thus, although influential population control advocacy and Malthusian ideology during the twentieth century played a role in the legitimization and medicalization of contraception as a form of family planning, a line was drawn to exclude sex selective abortion.

A US climate in which the medicalization of abortion was tenuous at best thus combined with an international climate in the 1990s that was beginning to recognize the scale of sex selective abortion. Scientists developing PGD and MicroSort in the UK and US within human medicine stressed that their application could avoid abortion by establishing desired pregnancies based on sex characteristics in the resulting child. As already described, British reproductive scientists vested in the development of PGD highlighted this feature to politically counter an anti-abortion bill that would have stopped research on embryos. In the US, professional bioethicists tentatively approved MicroSort for nonmedical sex selection if it could be shown to be safe and effective, justifying this position precisely on the basis of the technique's potential to avoid IVF and the creation and destruction of embryos (Ethics Committee 2004). "*Not* abortion" is a central feature of the material definition of both technologies. Boundaries drawn between ART and abortion, partially in response to local politics in their Western contexts of origin, initially drove a wedge between selective abortion and selective ART in the realm of reproductive genetics. In imagining lifestyle applications of sex selective ART, reproductive scientists deepened the wedge. Rather than taking their cues from the precedent of more long-standing sex selective abortion practices (Hvistendahl 2011), they disassociated their material-technological tools from the biopolitical contexts of population control and their related technoscientific practices.

## Unscientific "Low" Tech

In *Sorting Things Out*, Geoffrey Bowker and Susan Leigh Star argue not only that categories have "material force" but also that in their making, they create invisibility (1999, 3–5). One system created in the discursive formation of lifestyle sex selection categorizes technologies into "low-tech" and "high-tech." Most pronounced in the work of self-help authors, this system does three significant things in its constitution of lifestyle sex selection. It converges MicroSort and PGD together into the category of high-tech; it creates and validates the category of low-tech as a consolidation of all pre-conception methods that are not high-tech; and it fully erases sex selective abortion.

In high-tech sex selection, MicroSort and PGD are weighted equally as alternative methods. "Maureen's" ingender.com, Jennifer Merrill Thompson's book *Chasing the Gender Dream*, "Jane's" genderdreaming.com, and Robin Elise Weiss' book *Guarantee the Sex of Your Baby* all group together MicroSort and PGD as high-tech options. The technologies' common dependence on assisted reproduction, high expense, high emotional cost, and inconvenience are highlighted along with their scientific backing and accuracy. The "self-help" system of categorization minimizes differences between MicroSort and PGD, leveling the playing field between them, as the technologies are presented as options with comparable risks and benefits, or pros and cons. This high-tech category is flexible enough to draw in PGD alongside MicroSort, even though professional bioethicists maintain a distinction between them because PGD necessarily produces the problematic object of undesired embryos. The self-help system of categorizing minimizes PGD's identity as a genetic disease diagnostic tool, converging MicroSort and PGD into high-tech sex selection.

The high-tech category as described in self-help books and on websites (Thompson 2004, Weiss 2007, ingender.com, genderdreaming.com) includes the Ericsson method in spite of its questioned scientific validity. Ericsson's low cost makes it an attractive and more affordable option for self-help consumers who seek sex selection services from a laboratory outside the home. MicroSort and PGD providers would likely disagree with this designation and are even more baffled by the self-help community's other newly created category, "low-tech."

"High-tech" methods are contrasted with "low-tech" methods, sometimes also called "Natural Gender Selection Methods" (ingender .com), "Natural Gender Swaying" (genderdreaming.com), or "at-home techniques" (Merrill 2004). The self-help community, once again unlike the clinics, includes a range of nonscientific techniques in their system of categorization that can be applied at home. Their common convenience and privacy in comparison to high-tech and their low cost are highlighted. These include the Shettles method on timing of conception, its inverse, known as "O+12," and diets and methods based on astrology or the lunar calendar. Self-help authors do not deny that these methods have no scientific basis. They often underline that point. Yet they insist on their inclusion, lumping them together as low-tech, and they are open to the voices of some women who swear by them. One self-help author argued with her publisher for the inclusion of low-tech methods in her book:

> The low-tech was important to me because I didn't want this to be about money, and I think that we still need the ability to be able to exert some control over our reproductive health. . . . You're a grown-up. You can make your own mind up. *This may not be as accurate, but if it helps you feel you have some modicum of control, then that's fine. So, I felt very strongly.* [My publisher was] not as pro doing that. I convinced them that that was very important. (IF 10/20/10, emphasis mine)

In the tradition of classic self-help women's health advocacy, this author's refusal to deny "low-tech" a place alongside "high-tech" interventions reflects her understanding that low-tech may provide women users with "some modicum of control" over the process. Based on women's experiences with the medicalization of pregnancy, self-help authors rarely tout technoscientific interventions without any reservation. Their stake in the recognition of low-tech lies in acknowledging that "high-tech" often is experienced by women as handing oneself or one's body over to science, thereby ceding control.

Scientists and clinicians, on the other hand, may have expected that the advent of scientifically proven methods of sex selection would eliminate the use and spreading of, in their view, "old wives' tales." Yet, these methods have experienced a renaissance of sorts—newly validated as "natural," "alternative," or at least an option among today's techniques. Significantly, they are not represented by the self-help community as "backward." The scientific director of the MicroSort trial reacted to this development:

> One of the things that is frustrating to me is reading on the internet over and over and over and over again—they appear to be blogs about, but I think they're thinly veiled advertisements for Chinese lunar calendar for having your girl baby or your boy baby, natural methods for gender selection, that sort of stuff. Pretty much tired retreads of the same old thing that just don't work. As a scientist I find that very frustrating. I cringe when I see references to swaying and that kind of thing, because I know that people are wasting their time. Fifty percent of the time they'll be successful, and that sort of success, which is not doing it the old-fashioned way, perpetuates that sort of hope. (IF 12/8/10–12/22/10)

Much to the chagrin of scientists like him, both "Jane" and Jennifer Merrill Thompson argued that "low-tech" methods would never go away; "Jane" further asserted the existence of clear ties between those in the larger "swaying community" and that smaller subset that go for "high-tech." Some users want to experiment with low-tech for a while and then decide to go high-tech, she explained, and some who have had failed attempts at high-tech report going "natural" again, which can also mean that they take their 50:50 chances by just trying to get pregnant (outside of a clinic) without even low-tech interventions. One self-help author similarly recounts cases in her on-line blog where users choose high tech even after successfully attempting low-tech because they are getting older, cannot afford to have many more children, and cannot "chance it." Thus, self-help authors represent high-tech and low-tech as different ends of a continuum rather than sharply divided, mutually exclusive categories. Yet, as inclusive and comprehensive as the continuum appears to be, it reinforces the invisibility of sex selective abortion.

Significantly, the alternative to high-tech is a wide range of low-tech options, but not sex selective abortion. The system excludes sex selective abortion, "othering" it as a "drastic measure" that someone experiencing "extreme gender disappointment" might take. Often conflated with "sex selection," sex selective abortion is represented as a "backward" cultural practice when mentioned at all, reinforcing its illegitimacy. Sex selective abortion is eliminated often by lumping it together with infanticide as an antiquated, exotic cultural practice. Jennifer M. Thompson writes, "In places such as China and India, a boy baby historically has brought joy; a girl baby, the opposite, and sometimes selective abortion or infanticide has, tragically, resulted" (Thompson 2004, 11). One self-help author, reflecting on why her book content excludes sex selective abortion, stated: "In the historical perspective, and woven in several places in the book—not directly addressed—is the issue of sex selective abortion and infanticide. . . . I felt like the issue of abortion particularly for sex selection [pause] this book was divisive enough on its own. So, I chose not to really focus on that issue" (IF 10/20/10). When self-help authors mention sex selective abortion at all, they mark it as something historical or culturally foreign that does not belong within the temporal and spatial Western frame of lifestyle sex selection. Their erasure of sex selective abortion as a category of sex selection denies the relative contemporaneousness of ultrasound and amniocentesis (especially in comparison to some of the recognized low-tech methods in this system, such as the Chinese lunar calendar). It also denies that sex selective abortions occur unrestricted by geopolitical, cultural, religious, or ethnic boundaries in the United States (Puri et al. 2011, Hvistendahl 2011, Almond and Edlund 2008).

As Bowker and Star contend, "Each category valorizes some point of view and silences another" (1999, 5). Importantly, the safe, self-help spaces of lifestyle sex selection discursively assert new technologies of the self and the social. However, they create value not in a vacuum, but over and in relation to something else: that which is glaringly absent. The discursive constitution of lifestyle sex selection through new terms and categories is the constitution of a hierarchy that distinguishes between good and bad sex selection practices.

## The Transnational Biomedicalization of Sex Selective ART

MicroSort and PGD became acceptable in the fulfillment of a lifestyle desire for specifically sexed children through a multistage process of biomedicalization. Developed for use in the livestock industry, their application in human medicine required scientists to first articulate a justification based on prevention of genetic disease and avoidance of abortion. A distinct geopolitical, transatlantic connection, particularly among UK and US scientists in conversation with one another, provided the springboard for the subsequent meaning-making shift. The resulting composite, focused as it is on desire, lifestyle, and family composition, extended rather quickly the application of MicroSort and PGD to "family balancing."

While the local anti-abortion context in the US and the UK influenced the material-discursive development of both PGD and MicroSort, the international condemnation of sex selective abortion in the mid-1990s, connected as it was to critiques of abusive global population control policies, amplified meaning-making transitions in the biomedicalization process via implicit dis-identification. Here, I underline that requisite to the formation of lifestyle sex selection were countervailing ideas stemming from a preexisting global—the international population order wedded to development regimes. Following the anticipation by scientists of lifestyle selection, professional bioethicists would later make explicit that sex selective ART not only was not abortion, but also not China, not India, not family limitation, and not a manifestation of sex bias.

The meaning-making shift that occurred through the biomedicalization of sex selective ART took place within sites and through "techno-social" practices grounded in the UK and US. The overlapping domains in which PGD and MicroSort embed, ART and reproductive genetics, strongly associate with "high" science, the pioneering field of human biotechnology, and wealthy world regions, even as ART proliferates increasingly beyond those (Western) locations.[8] ART provides PGD and MicroSort not only with an *institutional* home, but also with associative meaning. As ART-embedded technologies, PGD and MicroSort gain definition through belonging and situation on the privileged side in a dichotomized world of reproductive technologies alongside valued reproduction, conceptive technologies, and neoliberal governmentality. Referencing Taylorist forms of modern industrial, assembly-line production associated with the automobile, sociologist Adele Clarke notes, "While the modernist reproductive body is Taylored, the postmodern body is tailored," and she describes concurrent processes that enhance "control over" and "rationalization" of reproduction alongside those that "transform" or "redesign" bodies "to achieve a variety of goals," explicitly linking the latter processes to "conception, (in)fertility, pregnancy, heredity and clinical genetics, and male reproduction" (1998, 10). Yet, I would argue that the idea of "postmodern" reproduction described by Clarke is not necessarily confined to specific technoscientific practices or geopolitical regions.

Like feminist theorist Inderpal Grewal's "transnational America," "family balancing" is ideationally global, able to "traverse" and "rearticulate" across national boundaries (Grewal 2005, 3). Cross-border applications of sex selective ART, as I will discuss in chapter 4, underline the institutional extra-locality of lifestyle sex selection—practices themselves sometimes transgress national borders through clinic networks. Cross-border applications rely on regulatory incongruences and the relative authority of fertility clinics to institutionally control practices within contexts of limited regulatory intrusion. While I explore the centrality of the fertility clinic as the site of governmental authority of sex selective ART practices in the next chapter, here I have foregrounded that a globally stratified system of reproduction not only gave rise to widespread practices of sex selective abortion but also prepared the ground for the biomedicalization of sex selective ART.

# 2

# Incorporating a New Technology of Hope into Fertility Inc.

## The Constitution of a Maternal Subject

AS DESCRIBED IN CHAPTER 1, SCIENTISTS, CLINICIANS, AND BIO-
ethicists involved in early processes of biomedicalizing sex selective ART
advocated its distinction from sex selective abortion. By turning to biopolitics in this chapter, I will reveal a deep connection between the two.
Drawing on Michel Foucault's notions of disciplining individual bodies
and regulating populations, I show how the maternal subject of lifestyle
sex selection formed across geo- and biopolitical contexts through cor-
responding, rather than contradicting, market-driven measures.

In *The History of Sexuality*, Foucault contrasts the ancient power of a
sovereign "to take life or let live" in his own defense with the era of "biopower" beginning in the seventeenth century, in which modern regimes
waged war on behalf of everyone and administered life by disciplining
bodies and controlling populations (1976, 139–140). In the enterprise of
administrating life, which involves the calculation and categorization of
lives in terms of political and economic value, sex became a critical target
of biopower for its access to individual bodies and populations. The two
main mechanisms of biopower as described by Foucault, the "anatamo-
politics of the human body" and "a biopolitics of the population," involve
operations of power that discipline and regulate bodies in both individual
and aggregate form. One of the most overt examples of a biopolitical
project in recent history—an international effort begun in the middle of
the twentieth century to stem global population growth—gave rise to a

proliferation of sex selective abortions. To understand the connection between abject and valorized forms of sex selection, I begin by expanding my frame to take stock of the neoliberal structural changes in state-centered population control that dominated the development agenda of the non-West during the 1970s and 1980s.

Lifestyle sex selection began to form concurrent major shifts in the "old" international population order, a structure relevant in the second half of the twentieth century that began to unravel during the 1990s. That order was characterized by several features, including international pressures on developing countries to control their population growth, centralized state population control policies, and numerical targets to reduce fertility rates, mainly via the proliferation of contraception and sterilization through strongly incentivized, if not coercive, means. Variations of this basic, state-centric, top-down approach existed in China and India during the second half of the twentieth century in spite of their different political systems. Since the 1990s a rise in globalization via neoliberal political-economics wrought changes in the system toward a more decentralized, market-oriented model focused on the individual. A "paradigm shift" prompted in Cairo by feminist activists who opposed both the language and the violence of population control buttressed this transition because it centered on individual women as rights-bearing, liberal human subjects. Rather than states meeting predetermined fertility targets, the private sector, both for- and nonprofit, stepped up to satisfy individual women's needs/rights/desires, which increasingly collapsed within market formations that took over the provision of reproductive health care. Concurrent with these shifts was the proliferation of ART in China and India as well as in other parts of the non-West (Knecht et al. 2012, Birenbaum-Carmeli and Inhorn 2009). I highlight this institutional backdrop in order to argue that the new terms, categories, figurative language, and visual images that produce the meanings of sex selection in the public imagination as practiced via ART are not wholly incongruent with discursive and institutional changes within a globalizing, neoliberal form of governance that came to dominate the arena of population and reproductive health policies all over the world at the turn of the millennium. That is, the relationships between pro- and anti-natalism, which have always implicitly undergirded each other, have become much more explicit. Although the biomedicalization of sex selective ART, as I argued in the last chapter, depended on its distinction from the population control contexts that gave rise to sex selective abortion, those contexts have simultaneously undergone material, discursive, and institutional shifts that complement and accommodate a global form of lifestyle sex selection via ART. Thus, even when sex selective ART remains illegal or unavailable in some parts of the world, it has become transnationally accessible at least to some streams of reproductive travelers.

Post-Cairo, scholars observed similar changes in China and India—the "state-citizen" relationship engendered during the old international population order began to shift toward "provider-client." "Providers" include a range of (often nonstate) actors, and "clients" are those who practice a particular global, market-oriented form of national allegiance. Public policy scholar Rachel Simon-Kumar describes concurrent structural adjustment policies in India that drastically reduced state spending on health and welfare because they were "not seen as vital economic activities that are crucial to market priorities," with a reorientation of reproductive health provision. Neo-Malthusian logics, she argues, continued to sustain this neoliberal economic agenda (2010, 139).

> By invoking the language of neo-liberalism, the state legitimizes the development of a "marketplace" of population policy. Thereby, the state could justify the emphasis on efficiency, opening up options that were not previously acceptable, such as encouraging private providers in the production, marketing, and sales of family welfare services and products, and cutting down services and subsidies. In principle, all of this was rationalized as being for the benefit of the "client/consumer." (148)

In a similar vein, anthropologist Susan Greenhalgh and East Asia scholar Edwin A. Winckler (2005) coined the term *Leninist neoliberalism* to describe the particular state-induced form of neoliberalization that emerged in China. China's population governance underwent a number of shifts, precipitated in part by the precepts of the ICPD program of action alongside neoliberal marketization (Greenhalgh 2010, 53).

> In the first decade of the new millennium, population governance has been a major site for experimentation with and adoption of new, more indirect, "human-centered" techniques of governance that have become the hallmark of the Hu Jintao-Wen Jabao administration (2003–). The embrace of such techniques . . . like the neoliberal methods of good

governance used elsewhere, work in part by promoting more entrepreneurial, self-directed private selves. (Greenhalgh 2010, xiii)

As fertility rates have fallen, preoccupations with population quality and family form have resurfaced alongside and in conjunction with the presumption of small families or singleton children. For the nation-state, women emerge as units of import, not simply for their role in the nation's development, but as consumers with needs and desires that the state/market should endeavor to meet. Greenhalgh clarifies that this regime change has moved from population control via "subjection" to "a more indirect form of control that works through individual desires and interests," centering a "self-regulating individual." She writes: "A critical shift is underway from individual subjection to individual subject-ification, which works through individual desires for such things as good health, citizen rights, individual choice, and small, modern families" (2010, 56). Simon-Kumar concurs, explaining in reference to India, "If duty and patriotism constituted the subtle rhetoric that persuaded individuals to participate in family welfare programs in the past, now it is the language of consumer empowerment that is being used" (2010, 151). Yet, significantly, both Simon-Kumar and Greenhalgh insist that these changes coexist with rather than replace the assumptions, imperatives, rhetoric, and even subjection of the old international population order (Greenhalgh 2010, 56; Simon-Kumar 2010, 145–146).

In this chapter, I argue that the institutional development of ART into a global form has occurred laterally alongside changes in the old international population order beginning in the 1990s. ART is no longer separate from, but rather is a part of that order, bridging divides between hemispheres and formerly separated biopolitical contexts. Fertility clinics make up some of the diverse, decentralized institutional structures of globalized population governance alongside private or state-run entities that parcel out contraceptives. In a particularly overt example, Amrita Pande, in her book on transnational commercial surrogacy in India, documents egg donation and surrogacy brokers working simultaneously as sterilization motivators for the state, or nurses encouraging women after abortion or sterilization to try surrogacy (2014, 109, 115). In a neoliberal and globalized population order, the compatibility of anti- and pro-natalist mechanisms increasingly reveals itself as they co-operate, sometimes via the same bodies. ARTs proliferate globally, including in the populous states of China and India, not simply as political means of reducing infertility toward pro-natalist ends (Inhorn and Bharadwaj 2007). After all, the imperative to reproduce frugally functions first as an imperative to reproduce, and second as obligation to reproduce selectively. According to National Family Health Survey data, the average age of sterilization for women in India continues to fall from twenty-seven years in 1992–1993 to twenty-five years in 2005–2006 (Singh et al. 2012). During a woman's reproductive lifespan, she could first comply with duty to the family and nation to produce children, then with the state's imperative of permanent family planning—yet still be young enough to provide viable eggs or a womb to the commercial market. She fulfills a duty of biological citizenship through contributions of not only public value but also bio-value to the state/global market (Rose and Novas 2005). I make this hypothetical point in order to demonstrate how formerly separate biopolitical spheres increasingly interconnect under the new globalizing regime of population governance, centered as it is on supranational markets and individuals. While I have argued that the biomedicalization of sex selective ART depended on its contrast to sex selective abortion and strictly separated reproductive contexts, the biopolitics of sex selective ART indicates their confluence. Beginning with the local institutional context within which lifestyle sex selection arose, this chapter highlights how the structural neoliberalization of the "old" international population order and the assertions of fertility clinic authority and protection of clinic autonomy from state intervention by various stakeholders in the United States do not represent structural contrasts or ironies. Rather, they are part of a continuum within a globalizing reproductive market that produces new faces of population control via the biopolitical refashioning of subjects, both individuals and populations.

In this chapter I examine the *local* form of lifestyle sex selection: clinical, state, and professional regulatory mechanisms and structures and the institutional context, movements, and texts in the US that gave rise to and govern sex selective ART. In chapter 3, where I explore the *global* form of lifestyle sex selection, I aim to show the applicability and embeddedness of this local form transnationally. Here I map the discursive and affective terrain accompanying the technoscientific development of sex selective ART practices through a variety of media such as statements by ethics committees, clinic websites, self-help books and blogs, and popular sources of news. Market-driven biopolitics construct four interrelated figurative subjects: the family balancer, the gender dreamer, the abject anti-citizen, and the global bio-citizen. Based on the liberal humanist rational subject of family planning, the family balancer emerged in tight connection to the gender dreamer, as subjects racialized white, nationalized Western, and yearning for a girl. These figures pose opposite the abject anti-citizen who is part of an oppressed population of women stemming from a backward, sexist society, slaves to their culture and tradition. Disaggregated from this whole is the emergent, individuated, neoliberal, diasporic subject or reproductive traveler who can purchase a trans-Western form of (temporary) bio-citizenship to share in biosocial exchange of gender dreaming or disappointment.

## The Self-Governing Fertility Clinic in Lifestyle Sex Selection

Depicted by legal scholar Alexander Hecht as "the wild wild West," the regulatory climate of US assisted reproductive medicine in the early 1990s lacked national funding sources and governing authority (Hecht 2001). Reproductive politics in general, and the contested moral status of an embryo in particular, prevented both federal funding and oversight of clinical practices and research involving ART (Ouellette et al. 2005, Adamson 2005, Hecht 2001). Health and human rights scholar George Annas explains, "Because it centers on babies and pregnancy and is fostered by the creation of extracorporeal embryos and the private recruitment of 'surrogate mothers,' reproductive medicine has proved impossible to regulate at the federal level in the United States and formidable to regulate at the state level" (2011, 459). Regulatory absence has remained a hallmark of US ART. Yet much institutional work goes into maintaining this absence of state intervention. To counter the image that anything goes in the "wild wild West," clinics proclaim that they self-regulate or adhere to professional guidelines on best practices. They sometimes point to the existing minimal oversight by some federal agencies over different aspects of their work environments, such as laboratory safety standards, quality control, and IVF success rates (Schuppner 2010). As bioethicist Guido Pennings asserts, "'No law' is also a moral position. Neutrality of the state is impossible here. A nation without legislation on bioethical issues supports the liberal position that every citizen should decide according to his or her moral convictions" (2004, 2689). Indeed, this position seems to have motivated the safeguarding by various stakeholders (the US government, the clinics, and others) of a relatively unregulated clinical ART practice. Many US fertility clinics operate in the private sector as part of a global industry that has grown out of reproductive medicine, a commercial enterprise that business administration scholar Debora Spar calls "a baby business" (2006). Lisa Ikemoto describes the role of physician-entrepreneurs—the professional corps that drives this institutional system: "Fertility doctors have not played the role of passive professionals surrounded by a whirl of commercial activity; many have become influential stakeholders who use a combination of medical and commercial practices to enhance their market positions" (2009, 280). Exemplary among these physician-entrepreneurs is Joseph D. Schulman, whose professional engagements indicate this trend. Schulman, for example, founded GIVF, contributed to the advancement of several technologies and methods in reproductive medicine, and has published a popular book on investing in addition to his scientific publications (Schulman 2007, Genetics & IVF Institute 2013).

## Vying for Control: The Case of GIVF

GIVF's application to the USDA for an exclusive license to commercialize MicroSort for humans exemplifies the clinic's tenacity in actively seeking control over its overlapping research and commercial domains as it committed the investment needed to bring the technology to market. The purpose of the USDA-issued license was to commercialize the government's invention, and the "most critical item" on the application requires the submission of a commercial plan, including "estimates of potential market size" and "profitability analysis" (US Department of Agriculture 2008). According to the US code of federal laws, the purpose of the *exclusive* license is to grant the applicant "a reasonable and necessary incentive to," among other things, "call forth the investment capital and expenditures needed to bring the invention to practical application" (Cornell University Law School Legal Information Institute n.d.). GIVF received the exclusive license in 1992 granted for the life (seventeen years) of the patent (number 5,135,759, dated August 4, 1992). With it, GIVF assumed *institutional* authority over the technology in the realm of human medicine. GIVF sought to demonstrate the technology's viability in humans for the sake of an explicit commercial aim.

When in 1993 the USDA granted GIVF an exclusive license to develop the USDA's patented Beltsville Sperm Sexing Technology for use in humans, it did so solely for the purpose of preventing X-linked disease. In 1995, GIVF asked the USDA to expand development of the technology to the *indication* of *family balancing*. Dr. Larry Johnson, a scientist from the USDA who developed the technology, recalls this moment. "One of their reasoning on it was, as I remember, it was that they couldn't keep the business going based on sex-linked diseases. In other words, there wasn't enough call for those type of situations that they could maintain a business. They had to add family balancing" (IF 9/14/10). A commercial intent drove GIVF's pursuit of the technology in the first place, and a commercial plan helped fulfill the criteria for GIVF's initial successful application for an exclusive license from the USDA. Yet, as a treatment to prevent sex-linked disease alone, MicroSort was not very viable commercially. The scientific director of the MicroSort trial explains, "The incidence of sex-linked and sex-limited disease is not that high. . . . we figured that the overall average incidence of all sex-linked/limited diseases [X- or Y-linked] is about 1 in a 1,000" (IF 12/8/10–12/22/10). Furthermore, from a commercial point of view PGD held a competitive advantage for the prevention of X-linked disease since it could more accurately than MicroSort select sex before pregnancy. Thus, *family balancing* not only provided a means to expand the market for MicroSort but also a way to keep it alive as a potentially viable commercial product. The USDA was likely not unsympathetic to this objective. From a statistical point of view, *family balancing* would allow the clinical trial to increase the numbers of subjects in order to more powerfully demonstrate safety and efficacy. Indeed, family balancing patients made up 92.2 percent of the 4,993 total enrolled couples in the trial between 1993 and 2012 (Karabinus et al. 2014, 6).

Nonetheless, the idea of family balancing was still strange, and Johnson did not expect the initial reception by the USDA to be favorable to GIVF's request. Once again, Johnson looks back on that moment:

> I was pessimistic. I didn't really have a position on it other than I didn't think the USDA would agree to it. . . . Dean Plowman. He was the administrator of ARS [Agricultural Research Service] at that time and he

made the decision. I remember the person who was handling it from the Office of Technology Transfer at that time. He told me, he said, he's not going to approve this. That was his view, but he was wrong. (IF 9/14/10)

June Blalock at the USDA OTT (Office of Technology Transfer), which handles all licensing for ARS, USDA, recalled the decision making. She clarified that the field of use on the license for genetic disease reduction was not extended specifically to family balancing. Rather, it was extended to all physician-approved human uses because the USDA did not feel that they should make decisions on medical ethics for human applications (informal conversation, December 21, 2010). Thus, the USDA in 1995 opened the door to the possibility of expanded indications for MicroSort while ceding institutional authority over the specific question of family balancing to the "overseers" of the clinical trial within human medicine, which at the time was only an institutional review board (IRB), not yet the FDA. Even though the USDA did not give family balancing a specific stamp of approval, GIVF likely interpreted the USDA move as a bureaucratic opening, especially given the general absence of federal regulatory mechanisms governing fertility medicine.

Before the FDA took over the trial in May 2000, GIVF made one of the most significant institutional moves in lifestyle sex selection. It established a policy that identified appropriate recipients of MicroSort on the basis of current family status, for example, married, heterosexual couples with an uneven ratio of sex among their offspring. Through its formulation of a "family balancing" *policy* (rather than only the invention of a new indication of use), GIVF applied a form of self-regulation. Rather than offer MicroSort to anyone, the clinic constructed self-imposed restrictions on who could participate in the trial in order to avoid practices that might be viewed as motivated by sex bias. By demonstrating prudence, GIVF preemptively self-regulated in order to prevent outside institutional intervention in its affairs. The clinic drew a line between the acceptable and non-acceptable as it asserted a nonmedical application of sex selection. GIVF's policy ruled out couples who wanted to choose the sex of their first baby or the sex of an additional baby that would not "balance" their offspring sex ratio. Yet, the policy required—and received—explicit approval by the IRB monitoring the trial. This validation coincided with the first of two institutional changes in IRB oversight. Initially, an IRB at Inova

Fairfax Hospital approved the MicroSort trial in 1993 for medical indications only. In 1995, GIVF formed its own, in-house IRB, which took over monitoring the trial and approved the "family balancing" policy (Wadman 2001). Thus, "family balancing" was a self-regulatory institutional assertion by GIVF as much as it was a contribution to emerging discourse. Accompanied by institutional action, change, and validation, the policy represents assertions by the clinic institution, GIVF, of its authority and control over the trial.

GIVF's assertions of authority and self-regulation in relation to Micro-Sort occurred alongside its initial resistance to federal regulatory mechanisms. For example, GIVF did not comply with the CDC's minimal self-reporting requirement on IVF success rates throughout the 1990s. Ouellette et al. (2005) assess GIVF's noncompliance in light of their venture to develop MicroSort:

> The number of nonreporting clinics documented by the CDC has decreased from 30 of 390 in 1998, to 29 of 399 in 1999, and 25 of 408 in 2000. While many consider it a successful reporting trend, a significant cohort of programs continues to defy the law by not reporting verified ART success rates. . . . One clinic, The Genetics & IVF Institute (GIVF) of Fairfax, VA, was listed as non-reporting in 1996, 1997, 1998, 1999, and 2000. This is especially disturbing because GIVF is a particularly large and well-known clinic. They have received national attention for pioneering the "Micro sort," sperm-sorting technology and advertise nationally on the Google search engine and in the *New York Times Magazine*. (426–427)

When the FDA first began to assert control over the MicroSort trial, GIVF resisted that as well, arguing that the use of MicroSort occurred within the practice of medicine, that it constituted an "innovative medical method, rather than a medical device regulated by FDA, but the agency was unwilling to alter its opinion" (Karabinus et al. 2014, 2). Ultimately, GIVF ceded authority to the FDA. GIVF then complied with FDA requirements, for example, by answering FDA warnings, ensuring quality control in its laboratories, and including trial data in MicroSort literature without making claims about the technology's safety and efficacy. In fact, the clinic's commercial aspiration for MicroSort had to be fully set aside during the trial since the FDA prohibited GIVF from making promotional claims and profit with respect to MicroSort. For example, GIVF had to ensure that all informational materials, including those stemming from collaborators in the trial, complied with FDA restrictions on labeling that prohibit commercial promotion of the experimental device. As the scientific director of the MicroSort trial stated:

> We have some regulatory lawyers that review everything that we write. Not only from a logistical standpoint it adds another layer of things that have to be done, it's expensive. In some cases it turns us, GIVF, the sponsor of the clinical trial into the bad guys. For example, we might come across just by chance a website of one of our collaborators that we believe in good faith has got something up on their website about MicroSort, and I usually am the one that ends up being the bad guy, contact them, and say no you can't say that. This is inaccurate, and I know that those words come from their media/advertising people, and not their scientific people. (IF 12/8/10–12/22/10)

GIVF faced further intrusions from federal authorities during the 2000s that impacted the institutional course of the trial. A 2009 letter from the FDA to GIVF's CEO, David Wise, warned of "objectionable conditions" and five "serious violations" that turned up in their inspection of GIVF's in-house IRB (US Food and Drug Administration 2010). The FDA also issued warning letters to MicroSort investigators Daniel Potter and David Karabinus, respectively, on November 2 and November 20, 2009, citing breaches of informed consent and the investigational plan (US Food and Drug Administration 2015a, 2015b). These may have precipitated the trial's move to Chesapeake Research Review Inc., a commercial IRB service company. Changing IRBs twice over the course of the lengthy trial reflected institutional changes in the life of MicroSort and GIVF. The first instance, in 1995, corresponded to a period in which GIVF held relative authority over the trial, but that began to erode by the end of the decade. At the time of the second IRB change in the late 2010s, the clinic faced several challenges to its control over the development and use of MicroSort.

In 2008 the trial officially ended after reaching its sample size limit of 1,050 babies, but through a "continued access" FDA protocol, GIVF was allowed to continue enrolling subjects while the FDA deliberated on the method's safety and efficacy. In 2010 the FDA prohibited continued access to MicroSort for "family balancing," limiting availability only to the medical indication of genetic disease prevention. According to MicroSort's scientific director, the FDA denied "continued access" to MicroSort for "family balancing" on the grounds that MicroSort did not fulfill a compelling public health need. GIVF countered that MicroSort prevents repeat abortions, which compromise women's health, but failed to convince the FDA (follow-up personal communication, June 27, 2011).

The second challenge came from the US Patent and Trademark Office (USPTO) when it declined GIVF's request for an extension of the patent on which it had held exclusive license for over seventeen years. The patent expired in August 2009; the USPTO granted the USDA a one-year extension on the patent relevant to MicroSort (5,135,759), but denied a second request because the USDA had failed to submit the request by a statute-imposed deadline. Thus, GIVF lost exclusive rights to MicroSort because the patent expired (personal communication with June Blalock, Office of Technology Transfer, Agriculture Research Service, USDA, December 21, 2010). GIVF sued the USPTO in the hopes of regaining its exclusive use rights to MicroSort, but lost the case in the summer of 2011 (Karst 2011). Thus, GIVF's experience with federal authorities can hardly be described as "hands-off" or indicative of regulatory absence.

Although the loss of its exclusive use license means that GIVF is more vulnerable to competition, the clinic remains not just a leading provider but at the institutional helm of lifestyle sex selection practices. It can do so because of the clinic's clear expertise over a complex method of sperm sorting by flow cytometry not easily replicated without substantial technical training. GIVF also preemptively undercut the FDA's authority by opening laboratories outside the US, that is, through jurisdictional circumvention (see chapter 3 for a description of the processes of MicoSort cross-border establishment and provision). Finally, by switching to PGD promotion, GIVF closed the void left by MicroSort in the US. Both GIVF and HRC Fertility, the two laboratory sites of MicroSort in the US, released newly revised or launched websites in the wake of the FDA decision to prohibit MicroSort for family balancing (givf.com by GIVF on June 15, 2011, and gender-baby.com by HRC Fertility on September 21, 2011). A switch to PGD as the prominent technology occurred under the banner of "family balancing" (GIVF) or "gender selection" (HRC Fertility) within these sites. In the 1990s, most fertility professionals, including those at GIVF, viewed the promotion of PGD for sex selection as unthinkable, but much had changed in the interim. Historically, GIVF had the capability to conduct PGD in its earliest years, but the clinic chose to pursue marketing only a preconception method (Schulman 2010). Most clinicians at that time could not contemplate the promotion of PGD for nonmedical reasons both because it potentially produced undesired embryos whose status was ethically contentious and because it compelled patients to undergo a relatively more invasive and risky procedure (IVF instead of IUI).

Compared to MicroSort, PGD fell outside the purview of various federal agencies of regulatory control. The FDA did not require premarket approval that would classify PGD as experimental and forestall commercialization pursuant to a determination on its safety and efficacy (Baruch et al. 2008, Baruch 2008, Schuppner 2010). The practice of PGD remains largely unregulated by federal mechanisms in the United States, and state mechanisms have only rarely filled that void (New York is an exception with regard to the fulfillment of laboratory standards) (Baruch et al. 2008). The far less regulated status of PGD, along with the material, discursive, and institutional convergences of MicroSort and PGD in lifestyle sex selection, created the conditions for a technological switch. US professional organizations stepped in to ensure ART clinic control over the decision of whether and how to apply PGD since it fell outside the locus of government or clinic-independent regulatory mechanisms that monitor safety and efficacy.

## Professional Association Texts: Devolving Institutional Control to Individual Clinics

In the absence of federal regulation of ART, national professional associations play a significant role in providing clinics guidance in self-regulation in the US. The texts they produce to guide clinics in the pursuit of ethical best practice can be viewed—as I will treat them here—as political instruments. The Ethics Committee of the American Society for Reproductive Medicine (ASRM), in particular, took the lead in the formative stages of lifestyle sex selection, releasing a statement on PGD in 1999 and another in 2001 on sperm sorting. The ASRM statements (1) recognized both MicroSort and PGD for their application in sex selection practices, (2) participated in the institutional convergence of MicroSort and PGD as a preferred set of techniques to those that require abortion, and most significantly (3) opened a door that authorized clinics to interpret on a case-by-case basis whether sex selection should be ethically permitted. After about fifteen years the association released a new statement in 2015 to replace the earlier two.

The first ASRM statement on PGD from 1999 begins by referring back to a 1994 conclusion it made regarding the inappropriateness of PGD for nonmedical sex selection, much like the UK's Code of Practice from 1995. The HFEA code, however, constituted binding law in the UK while the ASRM conclusion was an unbinding recommendation intended for fertility clinics operating in the US. The advent of MicroSort appears to have precipitated a return by the professional association to the issue of sex selection in general, and PGD in particular. Indeed, the timing of the 1999 statement came on the heels of the first media articles reporting the birth of MicroSort babies in 1998. "Since 1994, the further development of less burdensome and invasive medical technologies for sex selection suggests a need to revisit the complex ethical questions involved. . . . Among the methods now available for prepregnancy and prebirth sex selection are prefertilization separation of X-bearing from Y-bearing spermatozoa" (Ethics Committee 1999, 595). The statement recognizes MicroSort (without using its commercial name). The advent of MicroSort prompted professional institutional response and action on PGD. In this way, PGD's potential use as a nonmedical sex selection technique gained recognition *in relation to* MicroSort.

In one significant paragraph, the statement underlines a convergence of MicroSort and PGD as a preferred set of sex selection techniques: "This document's focus on PGD for sex selection is prompted by the increasing attractiveness of prepregnancy sex selection over prenatal diagnosis and sex-selective abortion." Inclusive of both MicroSort and PGD, "prepregnancy" techniques *converge* the two technologies in relation to less "attractive" forms of sex selection that involve an abortion, thereby validating some forms over others. The statement further notes that "the current limited availability of methods of prefertilization sex selection techniques [e.g., MicroSort] that are both reliable and safe" also played a role in the committee's decision to review the ethics of PGD as a potential alternative among more "attractive" forms of sex selection. It continues, "Although the actual use of PGD for sex selection is still infrequent, its potential use continues to raise important ethical questions" (595). Thus, as an institutional intervention, the 1999 ASRM statement confers recognition of a practical application of PGD for sex selection just as it institutionally addressed PGD with respect to MicroSort.

The text lays out a range of four different potential clinical scenarios ranging from patients choosing sex as a by-product of other, medically indicated, PGD services to undergoing PGD for the sake of social sex selection alone. It evaluated these from least to most ethically questionable. Acknowledging that ethical concerns sometimes conflict, the committee advocated for "ethical caution" in general, recommending that the most ethically questionable scenarios "should be discouraged," and the least "should not be encouraged." Importantly, the committee ruled out "legal prohibition" as an appropriate response, "because it is not clear in every case that the use of PGD and sex selection for nonmedical reasons entails certainly grave wrongs or sufficiently predictable grave consequences" (598). Embedded in the policy worlds of US ART, the ASRM professional association assumed its traditional advocacy position, which generally prioritizes access to technologies for individuals over government regulatory restrictions (Schuppner 2010, 449). In this way, the association ultimately conferred decision-making authority to clinics to weigh the ethics of sex selection on a case-by-case basis. Although ASRM recommendations are nonbinding, they nonetheless do institutional work by maintaining a status quo that discourages government interference while promoting practice guidelines that clinics can choose to follow, or not.

The 2001 ASRM statement on sperm sorting further widened the institutional recognition and opening to lifestyle sex selection. While questioning the scientific validity of other methods of sperm separation (such as Ericsson), the document recognized sperm sorting by flow cytometry (MicroSort) as experimental and as potentially efficacious for producing females, but noted that its safety and efficacy had yet to be firmly established. Just as in the 1999 statement on PGD, the text vehemently argued against policy prohibitions, but also against policies that would "condemn as unethical all uses" (Ethics Committee 2001, 861). As long as such methods could be found safe and effective, the statement reads, "physicians should be free to offer" them. It recommended "gender variety," which it defined identically to MicroSort's "family balancing," as "the most prudent approach" (863). In contrast to its ethically cautious approach toward sex selective PGD, the ASRM took on a more liberal stance towards sperm sorting because "it causes no destruction of prenatal life and is less intrusive and costly" than PGD (861). These presumed attributes of MicroSort depend on its coupling with IUI as opposed to IVF. The statement qualified its conclusions only on whether MicroSort could be shown to be safe and effective, but not on the ART method used, even though MicroSort used with IVF would raise its risk/benefit and ethical profile closer to that of PGD.

Taken together, the two ASRM statements, which the Ethics Committee reaffirmed for many years without change at regular intervals, *institutionally* constituted lifestyle sex selection. First, they recognized sex selective ART as not necessarily or always unethical. Second, the statements recognized individual clinics as the appropriate institution to interpret on a case-by-case basis, and without government interference, ethical sex selection practice. While the advent of MicroSort appears to have precipitated ASRM review of sex selective PGD in 1999, the preexisting interpretation of PGD provided the basis on which the committee could take a more liberal stance toward the ethical application of MicroSort. Indeed, the institutional constitution of lifestyle sex selection took place within the ASRM through ethical interpretation and comparison of the material dimensions of each technology against the other. Unlike PGD, MicroSort was labeled "experimental," but it was also characterized as ethically allowable for "gender variety" if found to be safe and effective.

The fallout of the two ASRM interventions was that they invited— even provoked—clinics to make their own interpretations. Just a few months after the release of the second statement on sperm sorting, Dr. Norbert Gleicher from the Center for Human Reproduction in New York challenged the opinion of the Ethics Committee. As he described to me:

And then out of the blue, the ASRM came out with an opinion saying that the principle of sex selection is acceptable via sperm sorting. And so it was the ASRM that really brought this to me and I think the profession's attention. I think most of my colleagues at that point were not thinking about ever using it. If patients came to us, we said this is considered unethical and *we said no, period, end of discussion*.

I could no longer say to my patients it's unethical, because our professional organization just declared sex selection is potentially ethical. . . . that immediately obviously raises the question of which is the most accurate method of doing it. (IF 6/3/15)

Dr. Gleicher wrote a letter to the ASRM Ethics Committee in which he argued an ethical stance backed by his own IRB that compared PGD's near 100 percent accuracy in determining the sex of embryos with sperm sorting's inability to isolate absolutely pure samples of sexed sperm.

Gleicher's challenge led to confusion and misrepresentation of the Ethics Committee opinion in the news. The *New York Times* science writer Gina Kolata (1998) reported on Gleicher's intention to immediately begin offering sex selective PGD because his question to the ASRM elicited agreement from the acting chair of the ASRM Ethics Committee, John A. Robertson. Appearing under the title "Fertility Ethics Authority Approves Sex Selection," Kolata's article publicly announced an institutional green light from the ASRM for sex selective PGD on the basis of Robertson's response to Gleicher. However, that response misinterpreted the consensus view of the committee as well as the gist of the ASRM statements. Robertson had published his own personal view that choosing the sex of children ought to be an intrinsic aspect of any individual's reproductive rights (Robertson 1998). Consulting with only one member of the Ethics Committee, Robertson wrote a response to Gleicher indicating ASRM approval of the ethical use of sex selective PGD for "gender variety," although the association had accepted "gender variety" as "prudent" only for the application of sperm sorting should it be determined safe and effective.

Five months later, in February 2002, Kolata reported that Robertson retracted his opinion, deferring to the consensus view of the committee, which upheld the 1999 statement recommending that PGD use solely for nonmedical sex selection "should be discouraged" (Kolata 2002). Yet, the upshot of Gleicher and Robertson's institutional interventions was the public display of debate on the ethics of sex selection, leaving confusion on the ASRM opinion, thus further inviting clinics to compare methods and develop their own interpretations.

## On Their Own Terms: Providers
## Self-Determine Sex Selection Practice

Baruch et al.'s 2006 survey of US ART clinics revealed a variety of approaches taken by clinics to the practice of sex selection. Some disclosed the sex of embryos to their patients in all cases, and some only when patients asked for that information. Some complied with parental choice on the decision to transfer sex-specific embryos in all cases, while some only for second or greater order children. Baruch et al.'s (2008) findings showed no dearth in the number of clinics that provided nonmedical sex selective PGD against professional guidelines that discouraged the practice at that time. The decision on whether and how to provide PGD appears to have been increasingly influenced by economic pressures. Two of my informants suggested that the willingness of clinics to provide PGD for sex selection increased during the economic recession starting in 2008. According to a clinic director, "A lot of the people that are sort of jumping on the bandwagon and doing it now are the same people that really were beating me up and had all these moral concerns about it five years ago, but now that the economy is lousy they need the money, they need the business" (IF 1/26/11). An embryologist from a different US-based clinic I visited also suggested that the promotion of sex selection services provided a means for his clinic to stay profitable even in lean economic times (FN 1/24/2011). An NGO director advocating in a campaign on the issue of sex selection confirmed this trend. "We have heard from enough doctors that they themselves are sort of ethically queasy about this except that they also feel the market pressures. Right? So, the fertility doctor down the street is offering it, so there is some pressure" (IF 10/19/10). The Center for Human Reproduction (CHR) in New York claims to have been among the first to commercially provide sex selective PGD in 2002. In a media blog posting on CHR's website, the clinic similarly claims that it "has, so far, not experienced the decline in IVF cycles reported by other centers" on account of the recent economic recession because of its diversified "special" services beyond the treatment of basic infertility, which include "gender selection" (CHR 2011).

Law scholar Nicole C. Schuppner, who argues for greater regulation of PGD in the US, contends: "Often ART providers decide themselves what procedures of ART to practice and exercise discretionary control over the application of practice guidelines and their interpretation. Substantive decisions, particularly in ART, regarding the 'ethical acceptability of certain practices' have in the past fallen within the physician's own medical judgement" (2010, 450). As she suggests, several providers preached the principle of "individual choice" and "reproductive freedom," but often conveyed these ideas just as much in relation to provider choice as patient choice. Speaking of ART physicians' reception of MicroSort, the scientific director of the US MicroSort trial said that its future provision ultimately depended on the "comfort level" of individual physician providers: "You show them the evidence, and you allow them to make their decision. What I feel they will conclude is that it [MicroSort] does work. It is something that if they feel comfortable doing it, that that's something that they could do" (IF 12/8/10–12/22/10). Repeatedly, informants guarded the choice of whether to provide or not as falling within the autonomous territory of the clinic. They suggested that physicians should base these decisions on their personal "comfort" or moral and ethical convictions. The clinic director who expressed dismay at ART physicians "jumping on the bandwagon" of sex selection for economic reasons stressed that the decision ought to be made based on their own "principle":

> I respect people who disagree with me if it's based on a principled
> approach that is really thought out based on some conviction that
> they may have. But, when you have somebody who was against some-
> thing, and goes on about how terrible it is, but now it's okay, you know,
> like all of a sudden it's okay, I don't like that. (IF 1/26/11)

Clearly, these "personal" decisions reflect those with authority within clinic institutional hierarchies, not the views of providers of lower rank. Some nurses I encountered in the field both during site visits and at a nurses' roundtable at the ASRM annual meeting, for example, described their own ambivalence to sex selection, especially when transitioning from working primarily with infertility patients. One nurse working at a clinic in the US Northeast who attended the nurses' roundtable on gender selection at the 2010 ASRM annual meeting described her feelings of "disgust" when a couple presented themselves for sex selection for a boy for inheritance reasons. She described feeling personally offended (FN 10/25/10). Another described at length the difficulty of transitioning from treating infertility to "gender selection" patients.

When I started in fertility, and I think I can speak for a lot of nurses, it was a huge change. In the beginning you are talking to these patients that can't have kids. Right? So, you have that mentality, these poor people, they can't have kids. It's very emotional, very stressful. And, then all of a sudden now you're treating these patients that already have kids, right? And, they're coming in just because they want to have the sex that they want, so you have a totally different outlook on the patient and what their expectations are when they come in. . . . It was a hard transition for me and a lot of nurses, and our embryologist too. She's doing something different than what she was used to doing, too. It was all about getting a fertility patient pregnant and starting a family, and now we're building on families that have already formed. (IF 7/26/10)

Leading the roundtable luncheon organized by the ASRM Nurses' Professional Group at the annual meeting of the ASRM in 2010, one nurse discussed patient counseling, support, screening, and consent procedures related to sex selection. The session seemed to mark a small but nonetheless existing institutional openness by the ASRM to providers' growing willingness to move beyond the ethical controversy of sex selection to face challenges associated with clinical practice. The nurse, for example, characterized fertile sex selection patients as having "high expectations" and being "determined, anxious, demanding, independent"; she described the infertility patients as "hopeful, grateful, dependent, needy, fearful" (handout of powerpoint slides to roundtable participants). One challenge faced in her clinic related to accommodating sex selection patients with children in separate waiting rooms with play areas so as not to offend infertility patients.

Fifteen years after the release of the second ASRM statement on sperm sorting, contemporary lifestyle forms of sex selection can no longer be described in potential terms. The evolution of the practice reveals the increasing inapplicability of the initial ASRM positions to real-world situations of lifestyle sex selection. Clinic directors have moved from discussing the ethical dimensions to addressing the commercial dimensions of MicroSort and PGD. For example, one clinic director who has largely promoted PGD in his practice admitted that MicroSort has a "draw" for potential users over PGD because of the relatively low cost of

IUI. However, since couples have to attempt IUI several times for it to reach the same rate of effectiveness as IVF, he argued, the expenses tend to equalize and the "draw" is "artificial" (IF 8/24/10).

Second, although MicroSort, unlike PGD, can be used with IUI, this combination cannot be presumed. Subjects in the MicroSort trial initially sought to couple MicroSort with IUI over IVF, but this has changed over time because, as the scientific director of the US MicroSort trial explained, "The people who enroll in MicroSort want a baby," and the success rates of IVF far exceed those of IUI. "The IUI-IVF/ICSI ratio [ratio of trial participants attempting MicroSort with IUI to those attempting it with IVF/ICSI] was running about 60:40, but recently over the last couple of years it has been gradually moving toward 50:50" (IF 12/8/10–12/22/10). Self-help author Jennifer Merrill Thompson, for example, wrote of her own experience with several failed IUI attempts before successfully attempting IVF. Thus it is possible that trial participants—most of whom attempted MicroSort on average three times (Darnovsky 2003)—gravitated toward IVF if their attempts with IUI failed. Given this reality, ASRM ethicists likely overidentified MicroSort with IUI, wrongly assuming users would always choose IUI when given that option.

Finally, changes in PGD technology now allow simultaneous analysis of all chromosomes on the biopsied embryonic cell. Results of a PGD analysis using micro-array technology will always include information on sex as a by-product of any application of PGD. In addition, most cases of sex selective PGD in the clinics I visited involved some form of a combined "medical" application of PGD such as aneuploidy screening (tests that check for chromosomal abnormalities) even when patients approached the clinic initially only for sex selection. Thus, in real-world practice, both the least and most ethical case scenarios of PGD for nonmedical sex selection as described in the 1999 ASRM statement apply. These include cases where the "patient requests IVF and PGD solely for the purpose of sex identification" (case scenario "d," evaluated as least ethical), but also the case where the "patient learns sex identification of embryo as *part of*, or as a *by-product of*, PGD done for other medical reasons" (case scenario "a," evaluated as least unethical). Thus, to the extent that PGD becomes a routine intervention in IVF, so does the option to preselect the sex of embryos. An article by the European Society of Human Reproduction and Embryology Task Force has recognized this potential, citing it as a reason to revisit the ethics and legality of "sex selection for non-medical reasons" (Dondorp et al. 2013, 1448). The line between nonmedical and medical applications of sex selection, which the ASRM attempted to draw in order to evaluate the ethical acceptability of sex selective PGD in relative terms, blurs. As a direct result of lack of regulation, practices move increasingly into a gray area of overlapping medical and nonmedical use.

Perhaps because it could no longer ignore these realities, the ASRM Ethics Committee issued a third statement replacing the first two, which, from an ethical standpoint, throws the door wide open for clinics to pursue sex selective ART in any form (2015). The statement's apparently inclusive title, "Use of Reproductive Technology for Sex Selection for Nonmedical Reasons," does not, however, include sex selective abortion. Not specific to either PGD or sperm sorting by flow cytometry, the statement acknowledges "reasoned differences of opinion about the permissibility of these practices" (1418). Documenting arguments both for and against sex selection via ART, the statement does not provide a consensus view, instead urging clinics to come up with their own policies. Importantly, the ASRM has retracted its previous directive for clinics either to discourage or not encourage sex selective PGD for nonmedical reasons depending on the scenario in which it is sought (apart from or alongside other medical applications of the technology). While the statement concedes a lack of FDA approval of MicroSort, it also mentions over twenty years of use in animals and in humans abroad, suggesting that the FDA may, at least for some, not stand as the ultimate authority on safety and efficacy. This suggestion is further buttressed through the appearance of two scientific articles in 2014 and 2015 that present MicroSort as safe and effective based on US trial data (Karabinus et al. 2014, Marazzo et al. 2015). In the absence of an FDA decision on MicroSort, they reassert GIVF's control over the trial's outcome. The latest ASRM statement takes a "provider knows best" approach, removing any ethical obligation for clinics to provide or not provide nonmedical sex selection. It recommends that clinics allow for conscientious objection by employees who do not wish to participate in service provision, thereby protecting the self-determination of even mid- or lower-level professionals in deciding whether or not to participate in the provision of sex selection. A subsection on social justice concerns without accompanying recommendations comes across as ineffectual, presented apparently only for its potential impact on the decision making of individual providers. In line with the neoliberal zeitgeist, the ethical principles of autonomy and liberty, as addressed in the ASRM statement, trump justice in a context where clinics gain commercially by offering a new service in a competitive market. In the following section, I discuss subject-making in lifestyle sex selection through the elaboration of four biopolitical figures: the family balancer, the gender dreamer, the abject anti-citizen, and the global bio-citizen.

## Subject-Making in Lifestyle Sex Selection

Biopolitical projects involve the making up of citizens. Here I elaborate on the notion of the bio-citizen, described by Rose and Novas as follows:

> Activism and responsibility have now become not only desirable but virtually obligatory—part of the obligation of the active biological citizen, to live his or her life though acts of calculation and choice. Such a citizen is obliged to inform him or herself not only about current illness, but also about susceptibilities and predispositions. Once so informed such an active biological citizen is obliged to take appropriate steps, such as adjusting diet, lifestyle and habits in the name of the minimisation of illness and the maximisation of health. And he or she is obliged to conduct life responsibly in relation to others, to modulate decisions about jobs, marriage, reproduction in the light of a knowledge of their present and future biomedical make-up. (2005, 451)

These citizens contribute both public value to states and bio-value to markets (445–448). Lifestyle sex selection transforms the potential interpretation of "acts of choice" in sex selective reproduction from one of ethical treason by an anti-citizen to a bio-valuable product of an "ethical pioneer" or "active" global biological citizen as conceptualized by Rose and Novas (450, 459). Below I elaborate on four biopolitical figurations traced by various actors, including medical professionals, self-help authors and patient groups, bioethicists, journalists, and entrepreneurs involved in the making up of an active biological citizenry of lifestyle sex selection. I employ a typology that separates these figurations for heuristic purposes, but they form as layers of the same representational strategies that ultimately produce longing and demand for objects that the market can satisfy.

## The Family Balancer

Journalist Kara Platoni points out the power behind the term *family balancing*, citing feminist theorist of reproductive technology Charis Thompson:

> The genius of the term "family balancing" lies in its ability to transform a social anxiety (desire for a boy or a girl) into a clinical diagnosis with a recommended medical solution. [Thompson] compares it to recently developed ideas about body shape "proportionality" that have become accepted as rationales for plastic surgery. "So if you have a too-small bust for a ratio to your hips, it's now a 'bodily imbalance,'" she says. "It's a medical concept—it's not that you're vain. That seems to me very similar to the rationale in 'family balancing.'" (Platoni, 2004)

Thompson describes a classic process of biomedicalization, when a social issue becomes an individualized medical problem. The term itself refers not to a pathology (medical or social) but rather to a positive action, a "balancing," holding implicit the subject of that action (the family balancer)—the one who technoscientifically takes action to correct an imbalance. In the same way that *family planning* became a synonym for contraceptive use that called on a modern subject to *control* her fertility for the sake of her health, her liberation, the betterment of her race (eugenics), or her nation's development (especially in non-West countries), family balancing calls on a postmodern, Western, or, more recently, (trans)Western-global subject to *(trans)form* her family for the sake of an individual desire, dream, or ideal. Family planning represents not only a practice but also a range of techniques that assist in avoiding pregnancy. Modern contraceptives were developed for mass-scale usage—not to treat a medical problem but to treat social and political ones, such as the feminist impulse of helping women avoid pregnancy or a nationalist imperative to control population growth. Family planning operated by *creating* the desire for smaller families as much as it *treated* that desire. Family balancing meets these criteria, and has similarly come to represent not only a practice but a variety of sex selective techniques that do not rely on abortion. Its innovation lies thus not in its total difference from the modes of operation and conditions of population control, but rather in the inherent tension that makes it both unlike and like sex selective abortion. In the overwhelming appeals to difference from sex selective abortion that have occurred within biomedicalization processes, similarities get blackboxed from view. Here I explore how the "family balancer" as a subject position lies at the crux of both biomedicalization *and* biopolitical processes by drawing on the politics of difference *and* sameness. It can be presumed that the family balancer is indicated for medical treatment because she refuses to have many babies to ensure children of both sexes. Her desires can be viewed as reasonable in part because she has already met the modern criteria for family planning.

Today, *family balancing* has come into wide circulation, even making its way into the tenth edition of the *Collins English Dictionary*, which defines it as follows:

> *family balancing* (noun)
> 1. (*US*) the choosing of the sex of a future child on the basis of how many children of each sex a family already has

Yet this was not always so. Having emerged within the context of the MicroSort clinical trial in its earliest years, the term has only circulated since the mid-1990s. Dr. Joseph Schulman, GIVF's founder and director, introduced the concept in a 1993 issue of the scientific journal *Human Reproduction* as part of "carefully defined conditions" that "would permit more ethically acceptable gender preselection of healthy girls or boys" (1541). At the outset, Schulman tasked the term with defining a new practice in relative terms, to signify something "more" in this case "ethically acceptable." From the beginning, then, the term was meant to produce meaning in relation to what it was not. It was *not* son preference, *not* gender bias, *not* abortion, *not* Eastern, and *not* even *sex selection* insomuch as *sex selection* was associated with son preference, gender bias, or abortion.

Both Schulman and Edward Fugger, a reproductive scientist at GIVF instrumental in the transfer of MicroSort to human medicine and in directing the clinical trial in its earliest years, carefully conceptualized the *policy* to deflect expected criticism. In her documentation of the early years of the trial, journalist Meredith Wadman of *Fortune* explains, "Fugger pondered how he might expand the trial without causing an ethical uproar. His solution was to offer the treatment to parents trying to conceive a child of the sex found in fewer than half of the family's existing children. . . . Critics could hardly blast the institute for opening an ethical Pandora's box: MicroSort would be correcting sex ratios, not skewing them" (Wadman 2001, 78). Years later, the term took hold among MicroSort and PGD users and consumer/patient advocates in online self-help communities. In their now taken-for-granted usage of the term *family balancing*, they often make explicit what GIVF only implied. "Maureen," an early user of MicroSort and participant in online forums at ivillage.com and babycenter.com, pioneered the first comprehensive website, ingender.com, to contain both self-help information and forums to share experiences and questions for those who desire a baby of a particular sex. In her "Gender Selection Glossary," for example, Maureen contrasts *family balancing* with *sex selection*.

> *family balancing*
>
> Using gender selection methods simply because parents prefer to choose their baby's sex, rather than medical necessity due to a sex linked genetic disorder. The term was coined to allay the stigma associated with "sex selection", which to many people equates to "boy selection" and the notion that one sex is inherently better than the other. "Family balancing" is meant to convey the desire of many couples, not to conceive the "better" gender, but to balance their families with children of both genders. (Ingender 2015)

"Sex selection" does not appear as an entry in the glossary, and the entry for "social sex selection" redirects to "See family balancing." Therefore, *family balancing* displaces *sex selection*, represented in this way as sex selection's socially legitimate form. Self-help authors like Maureen make explicit how the new term works to define a new practice against an existing "stigma-associated" form.

Part of the power and influence of *family balancing* can be shown through its travels outside of GIVF, where it has indelibly reshaped understandings of sex selection into a lifestyle form. Fugger et al. published a paper on MicroSort technology and the first births of MicroSort babies in the scientific journal *Human Reproduction* in 1998. Science writer Gina Kolata wrote the first news media report on MicroSort the same year in the *New York Times*. Her representation of the first MicroSort babies as a feat, or achievement, centers the reproductive scientists as subjects and presents the term *family balancing* as an artifact of the MicroSort trial. However, around the mid-2000s, news articles stopped attributing the term to GIVF or MicroSort, and the quotes around the term began to drop. A 2004 *Newsweek* cover article begins and ends with successful case stories of families with three boys who utilized PGD (the opening case) or MicroSort (the closing case) to have a girl child. The article defines family balancing as "the popular new term for gender selection by couples who already have at least one child and want to control their family mix" (Kalb 2004). Such usage reveals the plasticity of the term, which, partly through interventions made in news and popular media, began to define a broader set of "high-tech" technological interventions that include PGD.

The strength of the term lies not only in its generalizability with regard to methods used (as long as they preclude sex selective abortion), but also in its specificity to culturally Western contexts. Like Maureen, self-help author Katherine Asbery deploys *family balancing* explicitly as a way to demarcate a different (more legitimate and unbiased) form of Western sex selection practice. "In many nations in the Far East, such as India and China, there is an unnaturally high ratio of males to females. . . . When used for *family balancing*, indications in such countries as the United States, gender selection is widely sought without any preferential selection of males" (Asbery 2008, 76, emphasis mine). Elaborations on the term by self-help authors like these take for granted the meaning of *family balancing* as harmless. In an interview, the scientific director of the MicroSort trial reiterated the idea of family balancing as the policy of the trial, suggesting that this policy *by definition* and through its action ensures against sex preferences based on bias.

> Family balancing . . . I want to point out is sex-neutral. MicroSort does not do first baby sorts for family balancing. That is and has been a company policy. Yes, we do first baby sorts for genetic disease patients. Obviously. But for family balancing they have to have children and the sex ratio of those children has to be out of balance, and they have to choose a sort that will increase the likelihood of getting them a baby that is the underrepresented baby of that group. (IF 12/8/10–12/22/10)

Thus, GIVF represents the concept as a *policy*, a field of action that ensures through its very implementation against sex bias. *Balance* capitalizes on associations of evenness, equality, and even harmony to preemptively disassociate the term from sex ratio at birth *imbalances*, a phenomenon measured at macro levels of *population*—not at the micro level of the nuclear *family*. As the unit acted upon, *family* shifts the focus away from not only national populations (and their possible sex ratio imbalances) but also from *individuals*, whose isolated desire to have a girl or boy may be interpreted as indulgent or frivolous. *Family planning* similarly avoided associations of birth control with the fulfillment of individual sexual desire. By taking the emphasis off of individual desire, family *balancing*, like family *planning*, is code for rational decision making and a proactive action that one takes for the benefit of the family. Just as the use of contraceptives for family *planning* indicated responsible choice on the part of the user, so the use of MicroSort (and now also PGD) indicates the same for family *balancing*. In addition, like family *planning*, the term *family balancing* not only sanctions the decision to engage in sex selection via ART as rational but also constructs the social imperative to do so. *Family balancing* is not only rational; it ought to be done.

Yet, GIVF's family balancing policy in the trial imposed specific conditions to police desire at the same time as it structured a social imperative for heterosexual couples to ideally have children of both sexes. To qualify, patients seeking MicroSort had to be a married couple consisting of a man and a woman, had to "have at least one child," and to desire "the underrepresented gender among all of their children" (Karabinus et al. 2014, 3). Not just any desire for sex-specific children would do, but only those that occurred within carefully prescribed heteronormative conditions that recall the subjectivity of a family planner seeking to "complete" and ultimately terminate childbearing. GIVF's website explains, "Maybe you have three sons and have always dreamed of a daughter. Perhaps you have a daughter and desire a son to *complete* your family" (http://givfbaby.fertilitybits.com/familybalancing/, accessed on July 17, 2015, emphasis mine). Through its invention of family balancing, GIVF constructed the above social situations as reasonable (if not ethical) for the application of a medical technology. In line with a family *planning* strategy to limit family size, *balancing* becomes a reasonable means to "complete" a family. By drawing on the heteronormative conventions of the family planner—the desire to have specifically sexed offspring—became treatable. Looking back, the scientific director of the MicroSort trial speculated that the clinic probably restricted same-sex couples from participation at the trial's outset in order to increase the social acceptance of *family balancing* (follow-up communication, June 27, 2011). I would further argue that the core ideal of family balancing and gender variety depend on and reinforce strict binaried notions of gender and hetero norms even while, on the surface at least, their names appeal to the ideals of equality and diversity.

Since *family balancing* as an *indication* for MicroSort treatment is not dependent on a medically diagnosable condition, the inclusion criteria that qualified participants in the trial "diagnosed" the presence of a "reasonable" desire to sex select. Significantly, that criterion does not interrogate how those desires get produced. Individual desire, like the dominant freedom-of-choice rhetoric, can be stripped of the mechanisms that produce it, and thereby efface social problems or the social anxieties (as per Charis Thompson) that lead to those desires. Furthermore, by signifying rational desire as well as the ideal of a "complete" or "balanced" family, *family balancing* builds the imperative to sex select children—that is, it produces those desires just as much as it "treats" them. The marketing images of that ideal that appear on fertility clinic websites—a smiling heterosexual couple flanked by one boy and one girl—are the very same that accompany "small family happy family" population control messages in the non-West.

## The Gender Dreamer

In spite of its robustness, family balancing did not fully resonate with everyone. Jennifer Merrill Thompson, an early user of MicroSort and author of the self-help book *Chasing the Gender Dream*, recalls the initial strangeness of the term. Thompson became an advocate for MicroSort once she successfully conceived a girl after several attempts with the technology, after which she contributed to a MicroSort informational video clip on family balancing. Thompson recalls GIVF staff repeatedly prompting her to refer to her treatment as "family balancing," though it did not come naturally to her (personal communication, June 20, 2011). While *family balancing* gained some recognition in the *institutional* realms of clinics and an institutional review board for its pragmatic approach to defining a reasonable situation for sex selection, it failed to touch on the emotionality or morality of those situations. Self-help authors and users of the technologies, both online and in print, worked to fill that gap. In doing so, they constituted the figure of the gender dreamer. If the agent of family balancing still recalls the liberal humanist subject of family planning, the agent of gender dreaming has made the full transition to neoliberal subjectivity. Just as the state was obligated to meet the needs of the family planner to limit her family size, so the state/market is obliged to accommodate the desires of the family balancer in forming her family. Within the figuration of the gender dreamer, it follows that the market is driven to meet her desire for a particular imagined life.

More so than in the clinic, on- (and sometimes off-) line public cultures that have arisen in lifestyle sex selection allow users to express and have validated the feelings and emotions that surround the practice. Perhaps emboldened by the relatively anonymous spaces they encountered when meeting each other online, these self-help biosocial communities worked to reevaluate the goodness of the object—the "healthy baby" that is supposed to produce feelings of joy (Gibbon and Novas 2008). Among their neologisms, *gender dream* and *gender disappointment* gave voice to that which should not be uttered—explicit desires, fantasies, and dreams for a girl or boy baby and, its inverse, feelings of disappointment when facing the reality of prospective offspring of undesired gender. These discursive practices shaped lifestyle sex selection in a way that the appearance of new material technologies alone could not do. They shifted the affective atmosphere through the construction of new meanings and spaces intended to break taboos and create positive and supportive interfaces.

Drawing on Sara Ahmed's theorizations of affect, I interpret the work of these online public cultures as creating the means by which the technologies could become promising—by delivering the "happy objects" (a boy or girl baby) getting passed around in these sites, and accumulating "positive affective value as social goods" (Ahmed 2010, 35). "Happy objects," according to Ahmed, are not only those things that make us happy, but also things "evaluated and judged" to be good. Whereas *family balancing* could make sex selection "reasonable" or "rational," *gender dreaming* or *disappointment* that leads to the pursuit of a "happy object" (in this case, boy or girl baby via technoscience) could make sex selection morally good and socially worthy. Ahmed explains, "Groups cohere around a shared orientation toward some things as being good, treating some things and not others as the cause of delight. If the same objects make us happy—or if we invest in the same objects as being what should make us happy—then we would be oriented or directed in the same way" (35). In this case, self-help biosocial communities invested in the same object—sex-specific children.

Jennifer Merrill Thompson, a pioneer in the public culture that has arisen to create new meanings for sex selection and an early user of Micro-Sort, documented her experience with the technology in the aforementioned self-published book *Chasing the Gender Dream*. Thompson may have been among the first to coin the term *gender dream*, which put into words the emotions that went with the intention to sex select offspring. She described the intensity of the longing she had for a girl child:

> The drive to reach a goal—the determination to see a long-time dream come true—can be a very strong thing. It can occupy your everyday thoughts, it can shape your daily activities, it can become an obsession. It can make you do things you never imagined doing.
>
> That is what happened to me when I decided I wanted a daughter. And even as the months and years went by and it did not occur, and I gave birth to two wonderful, priceless little boys, my longing did not go away. In some ways, it became stronger. (Thompson 2004, 61)

The desire, she explains, stems from a vision of herself (the dream) that is inextricably tied to a vision of her family. At stake in the decision to "go for a girl" was her own gendered, maternal identity as well as her family identity. "I didn't want to be just a 'boy mom'—I really wanted to experience raising children of both genders. . . . I continued to carry that image in my head of a little girl posing for a photo, flanked by her two big brothers" (61). Thompson describes her desire for a daughter not merely as a preference, but as something far more deep-seated in her own visions and understandings of herself—not as an individual, but as a being configured through family constitution and other social ties. Other participants in these public cultures describe the importance of these imaginaries. Writing on the issue in the *New York Times Magazine*, Lisa Belkin makes public her own personal vision of an imaginary daughter named Emma. "I love my [two] boys fiercely, and I cannot imagine the world without them. But

I always thought—always assumed—that I would have a daughter. Emma, I called her during our silent conversations . . . I bought Emma clothes during my first pregnancy" (Belkin 1999). Like Belkin, others who have spent time in these public online cultures "out" their yearning for imagined daughters whom they sometimes name and for whom they (sometimes secretively) buy real clothes. Such maternal imaginings as described by Belkin and Thompson are imaginings of happiness in the future (i.e., they are anticipatory) and directed toward objects, in this case, a girl baby. Further, since happiness involves intentionality, as per Ahmed, "It is not just that we can be happy about something, as a feeling in the present, but some things become happy for us, if we imagine they will bring happiness to us. Happiness is often described as 'what' we aim for, as an endpoint, or even an end in itself. Classically, happiness has been considered as an end rather than as a means" (Ahmed 2010, 33). Thus, the technoscience of biomedicine as it extends its jurisdiction becomes a means of acquiring the "happy objects" related to self-actualization. Technoscience becomes instrumental not so much as an expression of personal liberty (or reproductive choice) but in the pursuit of "sociable happiness" (34).

The intention to reach out to others who feel the same way in a space where they will not be judged links members of these new public cultures more than shared experience with technologies. According to "Jane," author of genderdreaming.com, the large majority of online participants do not seek "high-tech" methods for reasons of cost or moral objections to IVF (personal communication, June 21, 2011). Users come to voice their desires in a space of acceptance and validation, to share ongoing details of pregnancies, to share ultrasound results and photos, and even knowledge on how and when to best determine sex in ultrasound images. Users also learn about and share ongoing experiences with "low-tech" and "high-tech" methods of sex selection, seeking solace when their attempts fail (either to get and stay pregnant, or when they face an undesired sex determination in a current pregnancy).

Self-help authors guard the ability of their audience to voice their desire for a baby of particular sex above all else. Thompson exemplifies this stance: "Although those of us who try gender selection understand that health is extremely important—and who doesn't want a healthy baby?—we also don't have to apologize for wanting something more, for hoping to influence gender" (Thompson 2004, 1). Belkin acknowledges the work done by repeated assertions for a desired boy or girl. Over time, she sees them conferring normalcy and social value to the object—"girl baby" or "boy baby"—without necessarily displacing the social importance of "healthy baby."

> These women do not question whether the sex of a child should matter. They take it as a given. Just as it is different being a boy than a girl, they say, it is equally different being a parent to a boy than a girl. Yes, they understand that the health of a child is most important, but that does not mean that everything else is unimportant. They talk about sex selection as if it were the norm, their right. And all their talk goes a long way toward making it so. (Belkin 1999)

Within these spaces it becomes clear that a boy or girl baby becomes an "instrumental good," or "object of happiness," and the technoscience of PGD and MicroSort makes possible not simply the fulfillment of a sex preference, but women's realizations of their imagined maternal selves. It is this emotionality that begins to explain the drive that motivates some women to make several attempts at lengthy procedures that involve risk and discomfort, if not pain, without any guarantee of pregnancy, let alone (especially in the case of MicroSort's relative lower efficacy) a baby of desired sex. Once again, Thompson asks,

> Why else would someone end up in the small consulting room of a nondescript building of an infertility clinic in Fairfax, Va., especially someone with no known fertility problems, speaking to strangers about the desire for a daughter? What could drive someone to subject herself to regular blood draws and pelvic ultrasounds, to clinicians poking around and checking her egg follicle sizes and the thickness of her uterine lining, to monitoring and reporting her sexual intercourse days—not to mention having to ask her husband to provide a sample of that most private of things, his semen, for a sperm count?
>
> Only a fixation that won't go away could push someone to do this. And for me, MicroSort was the answer to the unending question that seemed to rule my days: How could I make my dream finally come true? How can I conceive a daughter when it looked like my husband and I could only make boys? Everything I had been hoping for during the past

few years had led me to this place. And nothing behind those doors would make me turn away once I got there. (2004, 61–62)

Rather than a preference one can live with or without, gender dreaming/fixation/obsession expresses the intensity of the desires and emotions that drive lifestyle sex selection.

The interpellation of a girl or boy baby as the "happy object" that holds the promise of future happiness and self-actualization means its disruption can spell the inverse—"unhappiness," or disappointment. Ahmed explains the interrelated production of happiness and disappointment, whereby happiness as "an expectation" sets the emotional stage for disappointment (2010, 41). The mother of three sons, Asbery discusses her own gender disappointment as an embodied experience. "You feel like an outcast in your own skin," she writes. Gender disappointment is "one of those closet situations" and a "dirty secret" (Asbery 2008, 10–11). Similar to Belkin, Asbery imagined "Delaney," a daughter to whom she would write actual letters during her third pregnancy. Having to come to terms with an ultrasound result that revealed a third son on the way, Asbery puts into words her own feelings of grief at a "loss," once again making clear the intensity, indeed the very "realness" of the dream. She describes the moment when she learned the ultrasound result: "Oh, how could I explain [her crying to her two sons]?? I was crying for the loss of another dream. The death of a daughter I will never know. Crying for the sadness I felt for not having the one thing in life I wished for. Sobbing for my lopsided family" (Asbery 2008, 6). Similarly, self-help book author Jennifer Merrill Thompson describes her sense of a "void"—again, a kind of loss—that she felt compelled to fill. It is the sharing of these commonly felt experiences that draws women together in these communities. Through their interaction, they found language to make meaning of the emotions and embodied experience connected to lifestyle sex selection.

*Gender dream* and *gender disappointment* do not generally receive validation in mainstream public cultures; a self-help community arose to carefully guard a safe space where the feelings and experiences of group members can receive recognition. In this way they assert a shift in the affective atmosphere and work to reevaluate the goodness of an affective object, a specifically desired girl or boy baby in reproduction. Both ingender .com and genderdreaming.com devote a web page and forum specifically to this topic, and Katherine Asbery, a participant in the gender disappointment boards at ingender.com and babycenter.com, self-published a book on the topic, *Altered Dreams: Living with Gender Disappointment*. Although ingender.com does not provide an explicit definition of *gender disappointment*, it frames discussion by welcoming all users willing to abide by the following rule: "Rules for posting here: As always, be kind and respectful to all other members. Posts along the lines of 'you should just be happy to have children' are not permitted. (We already know this, thank you.) Unkind posts in this forum will be removed swiftly and without apology. This is a forum for support, not criticism" ("Gender Disappointment" 2007). More recently, it has added a space devoted to those with "extreme gender disappointment." Genderdreaming.com likewise acknowledges the diversity of situations that may lead to *gender disappointment*, defining both *gender disappointment* and *extreme gender disappointment* in the following way.

> *Gender Disappointment.* Gender Disappointment (GD) is the sadness that results in learning that your child is not the hoped-for gender. For some this is the mild disappointment that lasts for a few days as they adjust their expectations, and for others this can last for a significant amount of time as they deal with letting go of their dream of a son or a daughter and what that means for their family.
>
> *Extreme Gender Disappointment.* Extreme Gender Disappointment (EGD) includes feelings of grief and despair over a child's gender that seem to be unnaturally severe. Although a very small subset of those encountering GD, those dealing with EGD may be considering drastic measures to overcome the pain they are feeling, including: adoption, abortion, wishing for miscarriage, abandonment of their family, or even suicide. Although apparently and significantly disproportionate to the news of a baby's gender, those dealing with EGD often have past issues of physical, emotional, or sexual abuse, substantial loss, severe parental neglect or abandonment, or other markedly painful histories that have been associated with a certain gender. ("Gender Desire and Disappointment Defined" 2015)

The naming and defining of "GD" and "EGD" as mental health issues situates them as potentially medically recognizable categories. The site even points out that the American Psychiatric Association has not (as yet) conferred "official recognition" of GD and EGD as mental disorders in the latest edition of its *Diagnostic and Statistical Manual* (DSM-IV). The prospect of such recognition would mean that those applications of the technologies today deemed "nonmedical," "social," or "lifestyle" (as I have termed them) would be poised for another round of medicalization. Self-help groups present *gender disappointment* as a morally acceptable (Western) motivation to sex select as opposed to unacceptable (non-Western) gender bias, even though the "condition" as described pertains *in the same way* to the social and affective situations that accompany sex selection practice in the global non-West.

Self-help biosocial communities point to the complex social production of sex preference as a way of presenting desires for a girl or boy baby as benign. Such desire cannot stem from prejudice or bias, which according to this representation only manifests in certain (abject) cultures.

## The Abject Anti-Citizen

It should be clear by now that the family balancer and the gender dreamer, while distinct, are allied biopolitical figures—much like the family planner and the (sexually) liberated woman. While tensions between them do arise, they basically collaborate in the constitution of technoscientific identity-making because they rely on the same tools. The ICPD, as part of a neoliberalizing, political-economic global regime, privileged the individual over the state in remaking the international order of population control. The family planner's obligation to her family and nation receded in favor of the state's obligations to fulfill the needs and not tread upon the rights of individuals. Both pairs of figures—the family planner/liberated woman and the family balancer/gender dreamer—rely on and constitute a countersubject, the abject anti-citizen. In other words, both pairs operationalize a category of difference in order to constitute themselves. In the case of the family planner and liberated woman, this countersubject devastates her nation, family, and self with uncontrollable fertility. For the family balancer and gender dreamer, the oppositional "Other" resorts to killing female infants or aborting female fetuses for cultural reasons. Her status as potential victim does not absolve her state of abjection. It may even reinforce it.

The balancer and dreamer, as Western nationals, have biopolitical citizenship and are thus endowed with the power to represent the emerging practice. They exist, however, only in relation to "much of the rest of the world," or "China and India," and, in this way, the figure of the abject anticitizen is discursively always already embedded in her culture of origin. Readers of on- and off-line self-help literature do not see a figure of an oppressed woman stemming from a backward, sexist society, a slave to her culture and tradition, yet the numerous implications to a countersubject ask them to imagine her.

Narrative case stories in news and popular media, as well as the discursive assertions in self-help materials, project an individual woman, most often racialized as white and nationalized as American, who has strong desires for a girl. Using actual successful case stories made to appear representative, news and popular media delve into narratives of a woman's individual drive and always ultimate success in seeking an elusive girl after having several boys—women like Monique Collins (*Time Magazine* and CBS/*The Early Show*), Catherine Reed (*USA Weekend*), Sharla Miller (*Newsweek*, CBS/*60 Minutes*), Mary Toedman (*Newsweek*), Lizette Frielingsdorf (CBS/*The Early Show* and *Newsweek*), and Jennifer Merrill Thompson (American Public Media/*Marketplace*) (Lemonick 1999, Joyce 1999, Leung 2004, Kalb 2004, Morales 2002, Napoli 2006). Lisa Belkin's piece of long-form journalism discursively marks the nationality of these subjects as American by juxtaposing them against "much of the rest of the world." A highlighted line within the Belkin piece announces in bold, "Unlike much of the rest of the world, *Americans* do not prefer boys" (Belkin 1999, emphasis mine). Similarly, Perri Klass writes in *Vogue*, "There are countries, as we know, where the spirit of Henry VIII prevails, and everyone wants boys. And then there is the United States, where many of the most determined parents are out for girls" (Klass 2001). To the extent that images are included, these apparently representative *American* cases appear racialized as white.

Self-help authors flourish the subject with context and personality, underlining that in making and implementing the decision to "go for a girl," she is also self-determined, unlike her countersubject, whose choice for a boy is not her own, but imposed by others. Thompson writes,

> In many countries, women who bring sons into the world are honored
> and feted; it is considered a great accomplishment for the family. In the

United States, on the other hand, there appears to be more interest in trying to conceive a girl—maybe because of American women's increased roles and rights, their ability to say what they want and to "go for it," and they often want daughters. (Thompson 2004, 11)

Similarly, "Jane," of genderdreaming.com, asserted in a phone conversation:

> You do know that most people are after girls. The notion is as soon as you say "gender selection," people's minds go to China and India and the discarding of girls because they all want sons. Where *family balancing* happens where it is a legal practice—meaning mostly in the States, people like me, 90–95 percent are seeking girls. I am in a huge minority as someone seeking a boy. The perception is completely wrong. Completely. And the woman is driving this process almost 100 percent of the time. The husband has nothing to do with it other than being nice enough to go along with his wife. So the assumptions probably people make about the decision to do this, the process, and what people are after, they are probably wrong most of the time. It's mostly women that want daughters. (personal communication, June 21, 2011, emphasis mine)

In this way, self-help authors create a feminist script that links gender dreaming and particularly girl preference to Western civility and women's liberation. They make explicit women's self-determination and imply that in spite of her overwhelming desire for a girl, she would not resort to selective abortion. Often the desire for a girl is imputed to be devoid of bias, but just in case it is not, self-help authors take pains to repeatedly insist that desires for daughters are not accompanied by any devaluation of their sons. In doing so, they draw on an entrenched Orientalist and colonial narrative on infanticide as one of many "social evils" that justify imperial interventions. In a postcolonial era in which high rates of sex selective abortions are associated with the global East, the narrative resurfaces. In affirming their own biocitizenship and entitlement to practice sex selective ART, they assert that the subject-making of the family balancer and gender dreamer relies on the absent presence and alterity of the abject anti-citizen.

## The Global Bio-Citizen

Increasingly, as clinics target their marketing to minority populations and international travelers, and move to off-shore sites, the language of balancing, hope, and dreams, whose initial discursive assertions formed the (white) American woman subject desiring a girl, becomes prominent against the image of happy, "model minority" adults holding their desired babies regardless of their gender. Indeed, multiracial marketing, which produces visual equality while masking political dimensions of power and difference between these diverse groups, has arrived in lifestyle sex selection (see figure 2.1).

The family balancer and gender dreamer have taken on a global form just as the old internationalized figure of the family planner makes a similar transition in line with globalized, neoliberal markets. In her book describing changes in population policies in twenty-first century China, Susan Greenhalgh writes,

> As the first decade of the 2000s draws to a close, the deepening of marketization and consumerism is fostering new modes of reproductive subject-making and new kinds of global Chinese persons. Two trends can be discerned. First, China's people are becoming more globally savvy and ambitious, self-consciously making use of the resources of the outside world to produce globally superior children. In family formation as in other domains of life, there is a growing tendency for Chinese to see themselves as acting and competing not just on the national stage, but on the world stage. Second, increasingly, money speaks louder than state policy, allowing those with the means to circumvent the rules and find ever more exclusive and privileged ways of enacting their reproductive selves. (2010, 65–66)

In this way the shifts that have occurred in the old order, prompted in part by the ICPD, have laid the ground for the emergence of a new biopolitical figure—a trans-Western subject who traverses the globe in order to "enact their reproductive selves" (per Greenhalgh) by technoscientific means. Primed to enter globalized ART markets, this iteration of the family planner merges to become the new global bio-citizen of lifestyle sex selection.

# Gender Selection For Asians

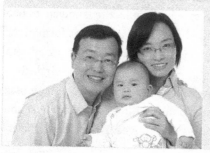

2.1. Monterey Bay IVF in California specializes in "Gender Selection for Asians" ("Gender Selection for Asians" 2012).

Importantly, the choice of boy or girl does not confer biological citizenship in these cases. Rather, an Americanized, Westernized, and assimilated status allows these subjects to come forward and claim legitimacy in their practices of sex selection regardless of where they come from or their sex preference. One clinic director described the emotional work of listening involved in serving traveling clients. With reference to patients from China, he underlines their need to explain their motivations.

> They're very different [gender selection from infertility patients]. You know, they're coming into something with nothing wrong with them, umm so the expectation is entirely service oriented rather than [pause] I won't say results oriented. In other words, they want to be coddled, and we do coddle them, and they want to be [pause] they're looking more for understanding, and legitimization of their motivations. Of course, we tell them in the consults you don't have to offer any excuses for this. It's available, but they all feel like they have to offer a reason why they're doing it. And, you know, we're happy to hear it, but it's not going to have any effect, on whether or not we're going to provide, because we do provide it.
>
> Yeah, I mean Chinese people come in, and again it's a real social taboo in China unless you're in the white-collar group. . . . And so they tell us, the typical thing is that we need to be able to pass the business along to a male, because it's almost 95 percent male out of China, so

they're explaining to me why it's gotta be a boy. I don't need to hear it, but I mean, I'll listen. (IF 8/24/10)

In part, the purchasing power of international clients affords them a temporary form of biopolitical citizenship that removes the strictures that would judge their motivations for sex selection immoral, if not criminal. To those who have the ability to pay and travel, the fertility clinic serves, in part, as a tribunal to hear testimony that will legitimize their desires for sex-specific children.

The cultivation of this category of subjectivity—the global bio-citizen— relies not on operationalizing categories of difference but rather sameness. One clinic director recounted a particular case of an Indian American couple going for a boy. His telling reconstructs the self-determined, this time "Americanized" rather than American, woman subject with powerful *gender dreams*, the "exact same story" as the legitimized racially white subject of lifestyle sex selection.

In the case of a Sikh couple I took care of, they are both second-generation people, pretty Americanized, as Americanized as you can be with the whole getup on and everything. Guy's a doctor, lady's a lawyer. He doesn't care. They have two daughters. He just wants to have another kid and is very indifferent about the whole thing. But, she, in her mind's eye since she was a very little child has always envisioned having a son and played through her mind model parenting this son, like when they were like four or five years old, played through her mind the sense of achievement, or kind of the praise, or whatever, the reinforcement that she would get from her parents, and from her in-laws, and from her family for achieving this. I thought that was really interesting. So, the women who want girls that are here in the states, or one of the British commonwealths, they, since they were little, when you talk to them, they give the exact same story, but it's a girl. The exact same story. They have, in their mind walked down the aisle, seen this person walk down the aisle. They have taken them to go shopping, taken them to ballet class. They have done all these things. Since they were very, very little, when they think of being a mother, they envision a daughter, so they really feel like this is something where they are really going to be sorry if they miss out on. (IF 1/26/11)

His insistence on the "exact same story" in comparing these cases aligns the sex selective practice by the Americanized Sikh couple with those of the dominant, white Western subject of lifestyle sex selection. Clinics, thus, have begun to discursively produce a global subject of lifestyle sex selection by transforming significant aspects of the still-formative white American subject into a trans-Westernized global citizen. Here it is not so much the rational "family balancer" but the "dreamer" that can naturalize the abject anti-citizen. As Sara Ahmed explains, "Happiness can function as a moral economy: only some scripts can lead to happy endings given that happiness is both a good that circulates as well as a way of making things good" (Ahmed 2013, 530). The political economy of ethics, which prioritized liberty and autonomy, combined with the moral economy of happiness, has the power to transform someone who might otherwise be perceived as the abject citizen (along with her bad sex selection practices) into a temporary global bio-citizen. These ethical and moral economies transform sex selective ART into a technology of temporary belonging in neoliberal times, while sex selective abortions become a technology of racial profiling and racialization.

In this chapter, I have focused on selected aspects of the institutional and discursive constitution of lifestyle sex selection that have occurred primarily within the US. However, I frame these within a context of globally occurring structural changes in the politics of population control away from state-controlled, centralized authorities toward privatized, market-oriented models in which the needs and desires of individual consumers take center stage. In this way, I demonstrate how fertility clinics function as arbiters of ethics and morality, as well as a gateway to engagement with new biosocial forms. As such they are part of (rather than apart from) transformations in the old international population control order, and they participate in the making of new forms of subjectivity that emerge in various sites across the world. Subjects relevant to the old order, such as the family planner, do not disappear entirely. Rather, they become the basis for new iterations of technoscientific subjectivity. In the next chapter, I focus on the globalized institutional mechanisms of cross-border sex selection in order to emphasize the increasing fusion, if not collusion, of pro-and anti-natalist mechanisms.

# 3

# Extending into a Global Market

Lifestyle Sex Selection as a Cross-Border Practice

IN THE SUMMER OF 2015 I VISITED GUADALAJARA, MEXICO, COORDI-
nating my trip with a team of US-based providers who travel to their satellite location there about eight times a year. I observed clinical practice,
including egg retrievals and embryo transfers, and conducted interviews
with the team, which included the clinic director and two embryologists.
I also visited the first MicroSort lab outside the United States, established
in 2009, several years before the Genetics & IVF Institute (GIVF) withdrew
its pre-market application for FDA approval of the sperm-sorting process.
In total, GIVF has been involved in opening five MicroSort laboratory sites
abroad, two in Mexico, one in Northern Cyprus, one in Basel, Switzerland
(for medical indications only), and one in Kuala Lumpur, Malaysia. While
GIVF owns the labs in Mexico, it sold and assisted in the establishment
of MicroSort in Switzerland, Northern Cyprus, and Malaysia; these sites
affiliate with particular clinics that hire staff to run them (IF 6/22/15).

In addition to interviewing one MicroSort lab technician and a "collaborating physician" (the director of a local clinic accepting MicroSort
patients), I had the opportunity to interview an unaffiliated embryologist
who had helped purchase and set up equipment for MicroSort in Guadalajara when it was first established, and who had worked in a Northern
Cyprus clinic in 2011–2012, where he estimated 70 percent of all IVF was
devoted to sex selection using a combination protocol of both MicroSort
and PGD. In this chapter I focus on transactions in the global IVF market
for sex selection where the US is both a destination for patient travelers
and a departure site primarily for providers who assist in extending the

practice into satellite locations abroad. I begin with a short vignette that illuminates the extent of these border-crossings in some cases.

On the last day of my visit to the satellite clinic in Guadalajara, owned and operated by a US-based clinic, I watched as two embryologists who had traveled from the US nervously prepared embryos for transfer. As the lead embryologist brought them into the clinical exam room, he announced "one male embryo for [name of client from Australia not present]" as he handed the catheter to the clinic director/endocrinologist, who transferred the Australian client's embryo to a Mexican surrogate. As the clinic director explained to me earlier, if a pregnancy developed, the surrogate would have to travel to Tabasco to deliver the baby since that is the only state in Mexico where surrogacy is legal, but the law did not stipulate that the pregnancy must begin there. The team brought with them six embryos for the Australian intended parent—four females and two males, but since only males were desired, the embryologists thawed both in case one did not survive. Since both survived, they refroze one and transferred the other. While I do not know the outcome, this one attempt at male baby-making involved a number of movements by embryos, providers, patients, and potentially also by the third-party surrogate both within and outside national borders.

Cross(national) border movements in sex selection are not well documented, although scholarship on cross-border reproductive practices recognizes sex selection as a potential border-crossing practice (Pennings 2004, Spar 2006). The prime motivating factor for cross-border sex selection is circumvention of legal bans on the practice, although unavailability of technology and expertise contribute to this trend. Sex selection has long captured the attention of bioethicists, who debate whether a non-medical application is inherently sexist, a slippery slope to "designer babies," a reproductive choice, or injustice (Dondorp et al. 2013; Dickens et al. 2005; McGowan and Sharp 2013; Purdy 2007; Seavilleklein and Sherwin 2007; Steinbock 2002; Robertson 2001, 2003; Wilkinson and Garrard 2013). While these debates do account for the differences that new technologies might make to questions of ethics, they have not considered the impact of reproductive travel now occurring for sex selection. Indeed, the acceptability of nonmedical sex selection for some scholars relies on a notion of Western cultural context that is discrete, bounded, and presumably immune from the harms that have arisen in non-Western regions of the world most often recognized as sex ratio imbalance in populations (Dickens et al. 2005, Purdy 2007, Dondorp et al. 2013). In this chapter, I focus on the cross-border form of sex selection, which I argue has important and as yet unacknowledged implications for ethical debate on sex selection. Any interventions to promote a more ethical practice must account for the webs of transnational practices highlighted here because they constitute the institutional means to decenter state authority and governance over sex selection.

The beginning of cross-border sex selection practices coincided with the emergence of regulatory inconsistencies governing sex selection worldwide. Bioethics scholars Wannes Van Hoof and Guido Pennings explain: "Consider the example of social sexing: the large majority in most Western societies believes that this is a discriminating practice. It is even considered a violation of human rights. Most countries specifically ban sex selection for non-medical reasons and it is only available in countries that do not mention it in their laws or where the fertility industry is largely self-regulated. This results in a current of people travelling for social sexing" (2011, 547). The discrepancy between an overwhelming absence of regulation in places such as the United States, together with prohibitions of nonmedical sex selection in China and India as of 1994, the United Kingdom since 1995, Europe since 1997, and Canada and Australia since 2004, prompt travel abroad to circumvent the law (Government of India 1994, Government of the People's Republic of China 1994, HFEA 1995, Oviedo Convention 1997, Government of Canada 2004, Government of Australia 2004). Like surrogacy and egg donation (practices also affected by legal inconsistencies), sex selection has become a cross-border ART practice. With few exceptions, most countries with legal prohibitions on surrogacy, donor egg IVF, or sex selective ART do not penalize those who evade the bans by seeking these services abroad (Van Hoof and Pennings, 2011, 2012).[1] Indeed, several legal or bioethics scholars view the extraterritorial application of law as undesirable precisely because of the contested morality of such practices. Pennings, for example, describes "reproductive tourism" as a "safety valve that reduces moral conflict and expresses minimal recognition of the others' [i.e., the minority's] moral autonomy" (2004, 2689). Pennings's view suggests that even states that, it would appear, do not stand to gain commercially from cross-border reproductive practices may still have a stake in their continuation as they provide a means of respecting the "ethical values like autonomy, tolerance and respect for other people's opinions" (Pennings 2004, 2689). ART clinics in jurisdictions where sex selection is illegal may also have a stake in cross-border practices for sex selection, as some discreetly participate in the transnational market either by accepting shipments of frozen sorted sperm to use in IVF procedures or by assisting in the start of cycles for clients who later travel abroad.

Since the founding of GIVF in 1984 and motivated by Joseph D. Schulman's frustration with the National Institutes of Health's lack of funding for IVF research, GIVF has epitomized the ethos of the self-determined private clinic corporation of US ART (Schulman 2007, 2010). However, its experience with sex selection demonstrates the tensions characteristic of a context of regulatory inconsistency. Initially, the unregulated institutional climate was constitutive of MicroSort's advance because it provided a "not illegal" space for new sex selection practices to form and gain definition inside the US ART clinic and outwardly through its website. By contrast, in Britain, PGD was developed in 1990 at the same time as the UK act that created one of the world's first state institutions (the Human Fertilisation and Embryology Authority, or HFEA) to govern it. One of the HFEA's mandates was to establish a code of practice as "guidance about the proper conduct of licensed activities" (HFEA n.d., i). Released in 1995, the third edition of this code prohibited the selection of embryos or sperm by sex for "social reasons" (HFEA 1995, 7.20, 39). Thus, in the very year that MicroSort in the United States first extended its trial to the nonmedical indication of family balancing, the UK's HFEA prohibited sex selection for social, or nonmedical, reasons. Currently in its eighth edition, the code today provides a more elaborated version of the UK's prohibition on sex selection. The first institutional recognition of nonmedical sex selection in the United States took place, therefore, the very year of the first institutional prohibition in the United Kingdom, creating a transatlantic dissonance in ART regulatory practices that provided an early impetus for the development of cross-border sex selection.

"Legal mosaicism" (Pennings 2009, S15) results in US clinics having an edge in global markets. According to estimates made by their directors, international clients made up substantial proportions of the total sex selection clients who presented themselves at two US-based clinics I visited (60 and 50 percent, respectively). The departure locations of these international patients suggest that many come to the United States or other potentially growing international sex selection hubs such as Mexico, Northern Cyprus, Saudia Arabia, South Africa, and Thailand to circumvent laws prohibiting sex selection.[2] In some cases, patient streams to the US originating in parts of Africa such as Nigeria, the Balkans, and Central Asia seek access to technologies unavailable in their locales (IF 10/12/10; IF 1/24/11, director of clinic A). Cross-border sex selection to the United States from other countries functions institutionally through an informally constructed and discreetly maintained web of networked clinics that facilitates the treatment of moving patients. Cross-border movements from the United States take place largely among providers through the operation of clinic and laboratory satellite locations abroad. These institutional formations foster movements of information, biomaterial, patients, providers, and equipment across borders, and together they make up the emerging global form of lifestyle sex selection.

In part, my motivation to study the global form of sex selective ART stems from a desire to disrupt the fiction of "crude geo-cultural divides" and the "implicit Orientalism at work," on which the constitution of lifestyle sex selection depends, especially within professional bioethics and mass media accounts (Whittaker 2011 612). Further, surrogacy and egg donation dominate the literature on cross-border forms of ART, and sex selection may add an interesting comparative example to the study of these flows. Small case studies have appeared that document Thailand and Cyprus as sex selective ART destination sites for travelers from Australia and Turkey, respectively (Whittaker 2011, 2012; Mutlu 2015). Having identified Guadalajara, Mexico, as a potential sex selective ART hub early in my study, I followed transactions particularly between the US and Mexico. My study exposes the informal and mundane aspects of a growing web of interclinical and laboratory transaction that realize sex selection across borders.

Ong and Collier put forth the term *global assemblage*, which welds together the implicit ideas of "global" as "broadly encompassing, seamless, and mobile," and of "assemblage" as "heterogeneous, contingent, unstable, partial, and situated" (2005, 12). They define "global form" as having "a distinctive capacity for decontextualization and recontextualization, abstractability and movement, across diverse social and cultural situations and spheres of life" (11). Knecht et al. distinguish various understandings of "global form" in relation to IVF. Among these, the production of "new orders of sameness and difference" and new universals relevant to humans such as "models of biological relationships among parts as well as wholes" (2012, 16–20). Lifestyle sex selection produces a new order of universal sameness in the construction of the global (unbiased) bio-citizen subject who transacts in a reproductive market. The new subject relates gendered individuals (the parts) to family composition (the wholes), or sexed sperm and embryos and babies (the parts) to the composition of their own identity (the whole). Yet, the transnational dimensions of sex selective ART occur via institutional assemblages that international documents ignore, alongside their implication in an increasingly stratified system of global reproductive practices. These clinical assemblages effectively decenter state authority within an international system that can only call states into account on agendas meant to address inequality.

## Patient Profiles as Transnational Subjects

Since my study did not include interviews of sex selective ART users, my own encounters with patients were minimal. I spent one day each at two US ART clinics conducting face-to-face interviews and shadowing directors (reproductive endocrinologists) in clinical situations that involved women in various stages of the process, observing one initial phone consultation with an African American woman, one monitoring of ovulation by ultrasound of a Nigerian woman, and one egg retrieval of a South Asian American woman. All of these sex selection clients were attempting sex selective PGD for a boy.

Having interviewed two US-based clinic directors in depth, including follow-up, I relied on their own accounts of their patient/consumers of sex selective ART. They offered a complex picture in which diasporic communities and transnational commerce figure prominently. Their accounts complicated the West/non-West binary prominent in depictions of sex selective ART in mass print and popular media. Immigrant and minority communities within Western contexts and wealthy patients traveling from developing regions of the world such as Africa, Central Asia, and Eastern Europe, as well as South and East Asia, clearly participate in lifestyle sex selection, but more often do not have the power to represent it.

One director described what he saw as two broad categories of patients he has treated:

> There are really two populations of patients. One population would be middle to upper-middle class or even upper class, females that are usually Caucasian, usually from some part of the British empire—Canada, Australia, New Zealand, England itself, even Hong Kong, and then the United States. It's weird that it's all British colonies, but that's kind of the way it is. I mean we do get some patients from other countries, France, Germany, and stuff, but not as many. These are women who are typically in their mid-thirties. They have on average two boys and they want a girl. So, that's one patient profile. (IF 1/26/11)

The next profile comprised mainly Asians (Central, South, and East) as well as some Africans currently residing outside their countries of origin, most often as first-generation immigrants in the West:

> The other patient profile is going to be someone from Asia, or Africa sometimes, . . . [It] could be China, not really Japan so much anymore, but sometimes Japan, China, Korea, India, Pakistan, some of those other little countries in there. . . . And then some of the Central Asian republics, they are not really religious people, so it's more of a cultural thing. But, they're like Muslims by heritage, but they grew up in the Soviet Union which was totally godless, so it's not like they're religious, but their heritage is still kind of rooted in those types of values, traditional types of values. These would be people that typically would be, if they're in the United States or Canada, then they would be usually first generation, came here to work or whatever, occasionally we'll see second generation, but not very many. So, first generation. (IF 1/26/11)

In order to avoid classifying these patients as having son preference, this director carefully protects their status as (unbiased) global biocitizens through his choice depiction of their "traditional types of values." He named Turkmenistan and Kazakhstan as specific examples of Central Asian Republics from which his clients stem. Yet, among this second profile, the director differentiates a subset—the wealthiest among these same categories of nationality that reside in their countries of origin:

Or if they're from the country itself, like if they're coming from India, or Pakistan, or any of these other countries I mentioned, they're not middle class people, they're not upper-middle-class people, they're like upper-class people that have a lot of money. People that own big companies, shipping companies, oil companies, computer companies. So, these are people that in their society, I mean even in our society, they would be wealthy people. People that are really high net worth people, maybe $30 million and up type of people. (IF 1/26/11)

The director estimated that about 50 percent of his sex selection patients come from abroad, mostly from Australia, England, India, China, South Korea, and Canada. It soon became clear that even more complexity undergirds these transnational routes. For example, he explained that a clinic in Thailand, owned by an Australian clinic, refers patients to him every now and then. Australian patients, who cannot for legal reasons access sex selection in their own country, may first travel to Thailand, and if their attempts at the procedure fail, they may then be referred to a US-based clinic. Indeed, news media publicized large and ever increasing patient flows to Thailand from both Australia and China, reporting for example that Global Health Travel, a medical tourism company based in Australia, measured a 30 percent increase (from 72 to 106) in the number of patients traveling to Thailand for sex selective ART from 2011 to 2012 (Westhorp 2013, Kaye and Jittapong 2014). A crackdown by Thailand's military government in 2014 on IVF clinics in the wake of a surrogacy scandal involving intended parents from Australia raised the expectation that sex selection would be declared illegal alongside commercial surrogacy. However, a Chinese press agency reported in early 2016 that it remains "an open secret in the industry that almost all the medical institutes that offer IVF services in Thailand" continue to provide sex selection "and the practice is still common" (Xinhua 2016).

In the second US-based clinic I visited, about 60 percent of the sex selection patients came from abroad, according to the clinic director:

The largest group of foreign patients come from Canada. Number 2 is China. Number 3 is England. But, we've seen people from every continent on Earth. A huge number of people from Nigeria, for some reason.

I think that's a combination of Nigeria having oil money and Nigeria having a huge problem with sickle disease. (IF 1/24/11)

When I probed for more information on other markers of identity, this director explained that the Canadians seeking his services were often immigrants from China, Armenia, and Albania. Four and a half years later this same director estimated that the proportion of his patients coming from abroad for sex selection had increased from 60 to 70 percent (IF 5/29/15).

As the director's comment portrays, a carrier of sickle cell disease in this case turns any patient into a "good" candidate for PGD, allowing them to legitimately pursue the method where it is available to screen for the single-gene disorder. However, this scenario does not involve the choice of sex as a by-product of a medically indicated use of PGD. Rather, the medical indication in this case provides a useful cover for and an opportunity to pursue sex selection for nonmedical reasons. Like the varied descriptions provided by these clinic directors of their sex selection clientele, Whittaker acknowledges that "couples seeking cross-border reproductive care are not a homogenous group" (2011, 615). In her study of cross-border sex selection from Australia to Thailand, she puts forth the idea of "reproductive opportunists, exploiting regulatory deficiencies and biomedical entrepreneurialism to purchase whatever services they desire" (615). Through the utilization of a medical application of PGD primarily for nonmedical ends, opportunists can also exploit the medical justification for these technologies. The opportunist contrasts with Inhorn and Patrizio's depiction of "reproductive exiles," a term they use to convey the "sense of betrayal and abandonment that most IVF patients feel as citizens of countries where their reproductive needs cannot or will not be met" (Inhorn and Patrizio 2012b, 510). With the stakes high in naming practices that can convey support or disapproval, medical anthropologists and sociologists debate whether or not to use neutral terms seemingly preferred by the profession, such as *cross-border reproductive care* or *reproductive travelers*.

Other scholars confirm the complex identities of sex selective ART patients who travel to hubs outside the US. Whittaker revealed patient profiles including Thai expatriates returning home (what Marcia Inhorn calls "return reproductive tourism"), non-Thai, temporary resident foreign expatriates, and non-Thai, regional citizens primarily from China, Vietnam, and India (Inhorn 2011b; Inhorn and Patrizio 2012a, 161; Whittaker 2012, 156; 2011, 613). With difficulty, Mutlu managed to interview what she describes as "highly fragmented, potentially disguised and extremely mobile" research subjects—travelers from Turkey to Northern Cyprus for sex selective ART. Most attempted sex selective PGD for a boy after having several girls, and Mutlu interprets their desires as tied to specific social anxieties and pressures that make masculinity achievable for men only once they bear sons (Mutlu 2015, 222). An embryologist I interviewed who worked in a clinic with exclusive access to MicroSort in Northern Cyprus in 2011–2012 recalled foreign patients predominantly from the UK and Spain in addition to Turkey (IF 5/29/15).

In Mexico, sex selective PGD users come primarily from abroad, most often from the US, then Europe, especially Spain, and then Canada and Australia (IF 5/29/15, embryologist). One US-based clinic director who regularly travels to his satellite location in Mexico said that once he began to advertise reduced-cost IVF services two years ago, his clients from the US to Mexico increased three-fold. Although PGD costs are the same, IVF prices go down by nearly $10,000 due to reduced ancillary costs such as use of the hospital in Mexico, which he claimed actually had better equipment than in a main city of his operations in the western region of the US (IF 5/29/15). Sometimes Mexico provides a convenient US satellite location for those reproductive travelers who have difficulties getting visas to the US, such as those from China (IF 5/29/15, director). Interestingly, the end of the US trial on MicroSort did not greatly impact the number of US travelers for MicroSort, which has remained constant (IF 5/28/15, lab tech). Some travel for MicroSort IUIs because they do not wish to select or produce an excess of embryos (IF 6/22/15). Others have tried PGD but did not produce embryos of the desired sex, and they hope that a combination of MicroSort and PGD will increase that possibility. In many cases, men (most often from the US, Nigeria, or Australia) travel alone to the MicroSort lab to provide fresh sperm samples that are sorted and shipped frozen to other locations (most often to the US) for use in an IVF cycle there. Although the MicroSort lab will ship sorted sperm to any clinic willing to accept it, some clinics go through difficult dialogues before deciding whether or not to accept the processed material, especially when they locate in jurisdictions where sex selection is illegal. One lab tech described a generic example, but pointed out that such requests often come from Spain:

> It's complicated because that's on the clinic's end. Initially they said, "You know what we cannot proceed, because it's sorted and we don't do gender selection," and then they went like, "Well, we don't do gender selection because it was PGD, because we don't want embryos left behind but since it's sperm and it's sorted, it's fine." So, eventually, we don't actually go into politics. It will depend on the clinic. If the clinic says, "It's okay, ship it," I'll ship it. (IF 5/28/15)

Since it may be more difficult to find local clinics in their respective locales willing to accept shipped frozen sorted sperm, Canadian MicroSort users tend to stay in Mexico to conduct a full IVF cycle. Similarly, European users of MicroSort stay for their cycles, often taking advantage of IVF tour packages to Cancun or Puerto Vallarta (IF 5/28/15, lab tech; IF 5/29/15, cryobank director).

As described in chapter 2, sex selective ART providers dealing with cross-border patients provide significant emotional labor in the process of constituting patients as global bio-citizen subjects. This involves confidentiality and a respect for their decision to sex select. One public relations announcement for "advanced gender selection" in Puerto Vallarta quotes the clinical manager promising "to unreservedly embrace intended parents" (PRWeb 2015). Treatment *without reservation* and respect for privacy is cachet in the medical tourism business, especially when operating in "ethical grey zones" (Mutlu 2015, 218).[3] It permits an interpretation of sex selection as a rational and legitimate reproductive practice, alongside other forms of family planning. Although the MicroSort labs in Mexico are situated among the burgeoning service and product providers to ART clinics such as cryobanks and genetics labs, they nonetheless have a surprisingly significant amount of patient contact, especially to those coming from abroad.

> We have patients who don't really talk to us and we have patients who talk about everything with us. . . . We have patients who eventually talk to us so much that they come pretty much after every physician appointment . . . they come after the appointment and see if the lobby

is open to discuss what the physician said, because we realized eventually that it's really a hard topic to find someone to talk to without a natural opinion about it.

Because of the way that the lab works—that we don't have a physician here, that we don't actually do their job, that we are not involved in the business—they feel like someone who actually knows what I'm talking about, knows what I'm going through. . . . But they come and kind of—in Spanish "rebotar," it's kind of like they reflect the information [from the clinic providers] with you, . . . and you end up pretty much just listening and they just want a confirmation . . . That's it, that's all they want. (IF 5/28/15, lab tech)

This technician/lab administrator referred to some situations in which she intervened to clarify information with clinic personnel or even advocate on the patient's behalf to ensure more adequate fulfillment of patient care needs, especially when she perceived a gap in understanding between IVF patients and providers due to cultural differences. For example, she cited the specific example of local Mexican IVF providers not fully comprehending the predicament of a single woman traveling alone using donor sperm who required help with injections as she had no one traveling with her to assist. By smoothing over difference, she intervenes to ensure a standard of care that creates a veneer of equivalence among users, particularly respect for lifestyle choice.

Mutlu documents the secret travels of Turkish citizens to Northern Cyprus, one of whom "took pains" to "perform a preferred (modern) identity" by formulating her desire for a son as "family balancing" rather than "son preference." She carefully distinguished her own desire from those who choose sons in the eastern part of Turkey, where "backward and patriarchal" motivations dictate a desire for sons (Mutlu 2015, 226). The combination of such patient "identity work" with the emotional labor by providers constitutes a new meaning of sex selection via ART that confers an equivalence or sameness to patients, regardless of their origin, their desired offspring sex, or where they seek services. At the same time these actions form a boundary to so-called biased forms of sex selection practiced by *others elsewhere*. This boundary work phenomenon is one of the particularly global, that is, "seamless" and "abstractable," aspects of lifestyle sex selection.

## Technologies Compel Border Crossings

How lifestyle sex selection situates globally depends on the material design that the technologies take. Their relatively immobile but fragmentary form leads to a porous, Western, high-tech practice in which the United States figures as a significant node of global flows of information, bodies, and biomaterials. Unlike technologies designed for mass use, dissemination, and transfer from developed to developing regions (such as in the global form of population control), MicroSort and PGD are comparatively immobile. However, their technological processes can be broken down in a way that allows provision to take place across multiple local sites through the border-crossing movement of bodies, biomaterial, and information.

The global form of lifestyle sex selection depends on design aspects of MicroSort and PGD that defy standardization and mass dissemination. Both technologies require a high degree of expertise, specialized instrumentation, and complex procedures to perform, which compromises the accessibility (and mobility) of each technology. However, the divisibility of the lengthy processes involved means that certain aspects of sex selective ART can take place in different locations or countries. The beginning, middle, or end of the process can be broken up. A single application can thus cross borders involving more than one clinic and lab, and more than one nation-state. In this way, contemporary lifestyle sex selection situates within a web of interclinical and interlaboratory practice that can span across nation-states.

Material-technological aspects of the MicroSort process and human sperm delimit the technology's mobility in a way that, until the end of the clinical trial in 2012, drove global flows of consumer/patients to its sites in the United States rather than the other way around. MicroSort IUIs require fresh sorted sperm because freezing depletes the already reduced numbers of sorted sperm. Therefore, MicroSort IUIs can only take place in close proximity to a MicroSort lab, either in or very close to ART clinics willing to utilize the method. However, the combination of cryopreservation (freezing) of sperm and IVF-ICSI (which requires only one sperm cell to fertilize an egg) enable a practice that stretches beyond the local laboratory site. Although theoretically MicroSort-IVF cycles may take place entirely at a local physician's ART facility without travel to a MicroSort lab, this would require freezing the semen sample twice, first for shipment to MicroSort, and then, after the sorting procedure, for shipment back to the local IVF clinic. Relative to sperm in other species, human sperm survives a freeze-thaw process well. Still, only half of the sperm in the original sample will survive (IF 12/8/10–12/22/10). Freezing-sorting-refreezing processes take such a toll on the material output of MicroSort that GIVF's labs recommend gating measures such as a semen analysis and test freeze to ensure that the sample is strong enough to withstand it. They also recommend that male partners travel to a MicroSort facility to provide raw, unfrozen samples for sorting so as to avoid freezing and thawing more than once:

> What we generally tell patients [pause] we recommend that they come here to provide fresh semen for sorting, because they'll probably end up spending as much money collecting, freezing, and sending multiple specimens as they would for a plane ticket here. (IF 12/8/10–12/22/10)

During the US clinical trial, this contingency produced patient flows to the US, but it now draws patients to MicroSort laboratory sites such as those in Mexico. A lab technician in Guadalajara described the expensive process of shipping sperm to and from the US in a nitrogen-filled tank that weighs about 13 kilograms when full. She calculated an expense of $900 to $1,500 to ship frozen sperm once from the US to Mexico for sorting. If the sample yields a low cell count, a second shipment might be required, and this does not include the expense of sending the sorted sample back to the US. Since it is often cheaper for US travelers to fly to Guadalajara or Mexico City, MicroSort recommends that male partners travel to its lab to provide fresh sperm samples. In order to accommodate men's work schedules, the lab stays open on Saturdays. Men are asked to wait a couple hours after sorting begins in case a second sample is needed to increase sperm counts, but they can often save on hotel expenses by taking the first flight in and the last flight out. Since Mexico City has more direct flights, men traveling alone may choose to fly there to provide samples for sorting that will ultimately be shipped abroad. Women IUI users, on the other hand, may choose Guadalajara, which is a city easier to traverse in shorter periods of time, ensuring more rapid delivery from laboratory to clinic, and thus viability, of the required fresh sorted sperm samples (IF 5/28/15, lab tech).

Male travelers to MicroSort still incur the cost of shipment of sorted sperm back to local clinics in their departure locations. A participant at ingender.com, "EllaJools," inquired about the experience of other users on shipping sorted sperm to the US in a post dated February 21, 2016. She posted the full costs of sorting and shipping sent to her by email from the Guadalajara MicroSort facility:

| | |
|---|---|
| MicroSort® Sort | $1,500 |
| IMI documentation | $400 |
| Shipping, Mexico-US | $350 |
| Shipping, US-Mexico (tank return) | $350 |
| Nitrogen and tank handling fee | $100 |
| Tank deposit | $850 |
| TOTAL (USD) | $3,550.00 |
| TOTAL (USD) after the tank is back and the deposit is refunded: | $2,700.00 |

A respondent to "EllaJools," mentioning that her husband traveled to Guadalajara the year prior, advised, "First thing you need to do is check with your [US-based] clinic, if you already have one, that they are ok with that, if not, find one that is" (Forums 2016). Since GIVF withdrew its pre-market application for FDA approval of MicroSort, US clinics have to decide whether or not to accept shipments of sorted sperm from abroad via a method once under FDA jurisdiction but never approved. Since the process of finding and using MicroSort is largely patient driven, US clinics are often first approached by interested patients. If the clinic allows a shipment, the MicroSort lab administrator will follow up and ask if they can be put on a list for patient referrals.

> I do ask the clinics [if they have accepted sorted sperm from MicroSort, if they are willing for MicroSort to make patient referrals in the future]. Not all the clinics want us to mention that they have worked with us. So when the clinic is willing, we ask them directly, "If a patient asks for a clinic's info, do you want us to include yours?" Mexico will say yes. The

US—half and half. Other countries—it would be like, "No. [I don't mind referring my own patients to MicroSort, but] I don't want walk-ins asking for MicroSort." (IF 5/28/15, lab tech)

Thus, MicroSort labs participate in creating and maintaining lab-to-clinic connections across borders similar to the binodal, interclinical webs that sustain cross-border sex selective IVF users.

Apart from the technicalities of sorting, freezing, and shipping sperm, the flow cytometers used by MicroSort are not very portable or simple to set up or operate and require skilled technicians. Cytometry textbook author Alice Givan describes the instrument as "complex," "unwieldy," "expensive," and "unstable and therefore difficult to operate and maintain" (2001, 11). Only three cytometers served the US-based MicroSort clinical trial. Typically, each MicroSort lab site outside the US is equipped with one cytometer and staffed with two locally based technicians. As to staffing the laboratory, the scientific director of the US clinical trial said, "You just can't pull a MicroSort lab staff person off the shelf and plug them in and say okay start the sort. It doesn't work that way" (IF 12/8/10–12/22/10). The flow system is fragile, and sorting requires constant monitoring by an experienced, trained cytometrist. The director insisted that technicians must never walk away from the process. As one lab technician in Mexico put it:

> And, we have to be looking at the screen the whole time. It's not running by itself. The thing is, it's a flow, it's a liquid going through, anything can happen. . . . If you get distracted, you could actually ruin the purity of the sample, and you will have to start all over again. (IF 10/22/10)

Her account of a typical workday included tasks such as prepping, staining, sorting, and sometimes freezing sperm samples, as well as paperwork. Adding a second sample for sorting on the same day required careful management of the procedural timetable in order to incorporate lengthy cleaning procedures and the physical separation of workstations to avoid sample mixing. Two samples in one day seemed to max out their current capacity of one cytometer and two technicians in the lab (which the technician indicated was outfitted to expand). Nevertheless, these current procedures hardly constitute mass scale use. In human reproduction, the complex and unwieldy form of MicroSort prevents easy dissemination and mass scale use of the technology, and thus it orients toward niche markets typical of lifestyle medicine. Six years after its founding, when I first had an opportunity to visit the GIVF-owned lab in Guadalajara, it had already begun to diversify its product line to egg and sperm banking as well as noninvasive prenatal blood tests (NIPT). The lab ships blood samples from women only ten weeks into their pregnancies to Chinese genomics firm BGI, located in Philadelphia, for information on fetal sex and chromosomal abnormalites. As an experienced conduit between clinics and laboratory sites that require shipments between the US and Mexico, the lab has grown into a multitiered supply and service company for IVF clinics, obstetricians, and gynecologists involved in cross-border trade.

Similar to sperm, embryonic cells biopsied for PGD move from clinics to labs. ART clinics remove and affix cells from embryos to slides (for FISH) or place them in capsules (for micro-array CGH) in order to ship them to genetic labs that conduct PGD analysis. In return, those labs send information about the embryos that informs which ones get transferred. While embryos either return to the incubator to continue developing after biopsy or are frozen, their removed cells become movable parts that will never return to the embryo. In the words of one clinic director, "All we want is the information from the nucleus of that one cell. So, you can ship it anywhere" (IF 1/24/11). The cells move from clinics to genetic labs, and information about them returns along those same routes.

At the time I began researching cross-border sex selective ART practices in 2010, the combined time for shipment, testing, analysis, and return of information on the embryonic cell extracted could not extend beyond a critical five-day period post–egg retrieval, after which embryos had to be transferred. Single cells were biopsied on day three after fertilization, when the embryo has about eight cells, and embryos were transferred on day five. Due to transition of PGD analysis techniques from FISH to micro-array CGH, PGD protocols have changed with cells (sometimes more than one) biopsied on day five or six after fertilization, and embryos are transferred on day six.[4] The time crunch for a fresh embryo transfer requires reliably prompt overnight shipping, and some embryologists in Mexico also serve as couriers, traveling across the Mexico-US border to safely deliver the cells they extract to genetics labs in the US. As one Mexico-based embryologist said, "Some embryologists, they take the biopsy and they travel with the cell by themselves to Chicago or Miami and deliver the cell by themselves . . . And the cycle hasn't started yet. So there's some pressure of time" (IF 5/29/15). Obstacles in the shipping process do arise. One US-based clinic director on site in a satellite location in Guadalajara described problems that arose due to a delayed DHL shipment on one occasion and a delivery withheld by Mexican authorities during the fall 2014 ebola scare. The director resorted to hiring "one of the girls at the hospital" in Mexico to act as a private courier to deliver the cells to a genetics lab in a major city on the US West Coast. This worked for a while, but his traveling team has chosen to simply take the cells back with them, which requires freezing embryos for transfer later on another trip to Mexico.

A major improvement in embryo freezing—cryopreservation via rapid vitrification techniques—has impacted IVF protocols as well. The way this affects cross-border application of sex selective ART is twofold. First, frozen embryos increasingly join other movements across borders (as happened in the opening case story of this chapter), and second, IVF cycles increasingly occur in a staggered way, extending the period of time between egg retrieval and embryo transfer. Embryo freezing eliminates the time pressure associated with fresh embryo transfers (which must take place on day five or six after fertilization), and with it the need for rapid receipt of information about the embryos via PGD. The staggering of IVF cycles not only makes it easier to freeze embryos without compromising their quality but also appears to improve pregnancy rates by allowing a woman to recover from ovarian stimulation, which improves uterine receptivity and increases rates of embryo implantation and subsequent pregnancy. For cross-border application, a later embryo transfer requires that either the patient or providers travel twice—once for egg retrieval and the second time for embryo transfers.

Access to PGD is similarly compromised by the expense and scarcity of highly skilled labor and laboratory facilities to conduct embryo biopsies and the chromosomal and genetic tests. For example, a Nigerian couple I encountered during a site visit to a US clinic had a referral letter (shown to me by the clinic director without personal identifying information) from a Nigerian physician stating that the patients had no access to a PGD facility. A clinic director from a fertility center in Nigeria explained to me in a phone interview that he refers his sex selective PGD patients to South

Africa and sometimes to the United Kingdom and the United States for the same reason. A physician from Nigeria participating in a roundtable discussion on gender selection at the 2010 annual meeting of the American Society for Reproductive Medicine (ASRM) likewise referred patients to the United States and sought a PGD-trained embryologist willing to relocate to his clinic (FN 10/25/10). Even an ART clinic equipped with a PGD laboratory in the United States had to shuffle experts and cells back and forth from satellite to main clinic locations because the smaller number of cases handled at satellites did not justify the expense of replicating the lab. As one clinic director explained:

> I mean these are highly skilled, labor intensive things that go on. So, to maintain . . . I go to [a different city in the US] every five weeks. I fly in, I do a bunch of patients, I fly out, and that's it. Same thing with [city in Mexico]. I fly in, I'll do thirty patients, I fly out. The time that I'm not there, I can't have somebody—a highly skilled scientist twiddling their thumbs. So, what I do is I bring the genetics team down with me, they do the biopsy and they send it back up here to maintain the laboratory. Because the laboratories aren't . . . I mean one lab can handle thousands, and thousands, and thousands of slides. (IF 1/24/11)

This director references a PGD lab in-house that was at the time conducting analysis via FISH, but his multi-sited clinical network now sends cells in tubes outside the clinic to a genetics lab that can examine all chromosomes via micro-array CGH. Even within the United States, restrictions in some states (e.g., New York) on the licensing of labs that can perform genetic studies on the tissue of their residents will impact the destination of cross-state border transportation of biopsied embryonic cells. PGD labs, as well as the embryologists who have the requisite skill and experience to perform these specialized procedures, remain relatively limited or inaccessible.

Thus, both the form and design of MicroSort and PGD defy the modernist criteria of standardized, mass-produced and distributed products such as the IUD or other contraceptives (Clarke 1998, 10). Both technologies involve highly complex processes that require specialized labor and equipment. Consequently, these complex ART technologies are relatively immobile. Yet, the divisibility of the processes involved fosters the movements of bodies, biomaterial, and information to and from laboratory and clinic work sites within "Fertility Inc." What follows is a description of transnational transactions that globalize contemporary lifestyle sex selection.

## Destination: United States

Since the lengthy processes involved in ART can be broken up into parts, contemporary lifestyle sex selection has developed procedures that can span across clinics, laboratories, and nation-states. Border-crossing patients who undergo sex selective PGD in the United States, for example, begin their treatment in clinics located in their departure countries. Only after undergoing mandatory testing, starting on fertility drugs, and getting monitored for ovulation is it necessary for them to travel to the US for egg retrieval, IVF, PGD, and then embryo transfer. In these cases, information such as ultrasound monitoring results flows prior to the patients themselves.

Similar to the "affiliations and partnerships" in cross-border egg donations, such as from Britain to Spain or Canada to the United States (Ikemoto 2009, FN 10/25/10), departure and destination clinics work together to provide a continuum of care for moving patients. Departure clinics offer preparatory services such as initial testing, administration of fertility drugs, and monitoring of ovulation via ultrasound. In this way, the time needed at destination clinics can be reduced to the clinical procedures that span from egg retrieval to embryo transfer. When patients abroad contact clinics in the United States for sex selective PGD, nurse coordinators direct them to their local clinics to begin the process. US clinics take measures to keep network activity discreet for the sake of departure clinics operating in jurisdictions where sex selection is illegal:

In London we've got some clinics, we keep them busy, but we're very cautious, we won't give the patients the names of the places in advance. They're not doing anything illegal. It's totally legal, they're basically doing ultrasounds for us. But, I don't want to expose them to that, because they're very valuable to us and if they shy off, it's a hard [pause] we've developed these relationships over years, and the understanding is we keep it low key, 'cause they don't need the grief. (IF 1/24/11, director of clinic A)

One departure clinic in the United Kingdom that openly provides and advertises preparatory treatment for sex selection that ends abroad also does not disclose the names or locations of destination sites on its website. The website explains in an FAQ section that "the initial appointment and preparatory treatments take place in London, however, egg collection, fertilization, biopsy and embryo transfer take place in another country," at an "associate clinic" and that patients should expect to be abroad for about a week (Rainsbury Clinic n.d.).

Given both legal restrictions and the disrepute of sex selection among some reproductive professionals, the process of beginning an interclinical connection for sex selection treatment is not always easy. One US clinic director who has his nurses interface with departure clinics before sending patients there described the process of approaching clinics for the first time:

> We'll approach a clinic, if somebody lives out somewhere where we haven't worked before. We call the local fertility center—"Listen, we're from the [ART clinic name], we've got this lady who wants to do gender selection, would you mind helping us out?" Ninety percent of the time they're fine with it, and 10 percent of the time we get cursed at. (IF 8/24/10)

A nurse working at a different US-based clinic further explained that upon first contact with a new clinic, she might not relay that the patient needing preliminary ART services seeks sex selection:

> They don't usually cause a big stink . . . A lot of times I don't put on there [the service orders] they're doing gender selection. They know they're doing IVF. IVF is IVF. They really don't have any business knowing unless the patients want to disclose. What they're doing with their embryos. When I do the orders, it's just pretty much, I need an ultrasound and estrogen on these days. That's it! (IF 7/26/10)

She further described ways she minimized direct contact with departure site clinics by communicating to them via the patient. In the case of sex selection, the need to keep things low key, minimize direct communication, and generally uphold privacy (both for clinics and patients involved, especially from jurisdictions where sex selection is illegal) impacts institutional arrangements by keeping them informal.

Within this global form, the United States serves as one key destination for cross-border sex selection, and US-based clinics act as nodes from and to which informational and patient streams transfer. This setup cannot function without the involvement of departure clinics, but the degree to which they knowingly contribute to a sex selection cycle and participate in decision making around pretreatment protocols is unclear. One US-based nurse clearly indicated that her clinic controls all aspects of a cross-border cycle, and the departure site clinic merely carries out their protocols:

> We follow up every day. There is no question about that. It's not like you send them to the [local departure clinic] and they manage through the clinic. The main management is through us. The clinic is just following the protocol that Dr. _____ is sending, but every single day that they have appointments or results, we go through that result so the clinic doesn't deal with them directly, we do. The clinic deals with us, not with the patient. (IF 1/24/11)

In contrast, the Rainsbury Clinic website (genderselection.uk.com) indicates that the clinic site in London, where UK residents can begin their treatment, has a hand in both departure and destination protocols and procedures.

US clinic websites increasingly market to patients abroad. The Fertility Institutes' website touts the clinic as "worldwide leaders in gender selection technology"; provides foreign-language access in Chinese, French, and German; and offers travel assistance to international patients. The website also offers a sample case story of successfully assisting a couple from Canada facing legal prohibitions in their home country. A website (gender-baby.com) launched by HRC Fertility on September 21, 2011, indicated by press release that it is solely devoted to sex selection. An entire page on traveling patients reflects their importance in sex selection commerce.

> While gender selection may be controversial and even illegal in some foreign countries, that does not prevent patients from coming to California and utilizing the gender selection technology. HRC Fertility makes it as easy as possible for patients to travel to California for gender

selection. We are extremely adept at working with patients remotely while they are being monitored by fertility clinics close to their homes. (Gender Baby n.d.)

The website further reassures international patients that they can begin treatment in their home countries and lists the tests they need to begin the process.

Test results get passed along the routes before patients even make their way across them:

First contact is usually is by internet or telephone . . . We've got sort of a form that answers most of their questions, tells them where the offices are. The big question is always, well can you work with me if I'm from, you know, Surrey, England, and it includes an answer to that, "Yeah, we work with local centers, we interface with them, *we can keep you at home for all but a week*." . . . And, once the consultation occurs, then we go through all the details. We have the local centers near them order the preliminary blood work and all the testing they need. We have physicians see them at home. Get a clearance from the physicians and off we go. . . . *We work with about 140—last time I counted—different clinics around the world.* (IF 8/24/10, director of clinic A, emphasis mine)

Once the testing is complete, results are faxed to the clinics in the United States. One nurse described the challenge of having to interpret test results in languages other than English. A director described the daily routine in the informational transactions taking place between clinics working across borders:

And, they fax us results, each day as the stuff is coming in. So, you get here four o'clock, we got faxes flying in from all over the world, and we sit down as a group. We do a grand rounds with the list of active patients, and I call out the orders for all those people, the nurses hit the phones, and everybody's given their instructions for that day. The next day we do it again. Get more people going. (IF 1/24/11)

After testing, patients begin taking fertility drugs in their home locales. Working across international borders sometimes complicates the process of accessing and beginning fertility drug regimens that kick off the ART cycle. A Mexico-based clinic director serving international clients said he sometimes has to order drugs from global pharmacies that deliver directly to a patient's residence because such pharmacies have more flexible registration requirements for the doctors who place orders (IF 11/19/10). Similarly, "Jane," the author of genderdreaming.com, said that participants within private international forums on her website relay self-help advice to one another on how to access fertility drugs that start off their treatment cycles (personal communication, June 21, 2011).

Once the patient has several maturing follicles, she travels to the destination location for the procedural aspects of the treatment—egg retrieval, IVF, PGD, and then embryo transfer, all of which take place in less than two weeks in an un-staggered cycle. One nurse described that process from start to finish:

> So what I usually do is send to the patient all of their testing information like all the tests they have to do and I'll look up some clinics, *'cause now with me doing this I know some clinics from all over the world*, so I'll just send them, "This is your local clinic, I know this coordinator there, just give her a call, they'll get you in for your testing." And so we make the testing happen. Once we get the testing back, Dr. ____ will review those results and make me out a plan of treatment for the patient, and then what I do I make the patient a schedule according to whatever dates they want to be here for their vacation, or whatever, *'cause they're here for about twelve days* when they go through the process. So, they start in the country or the city that they are in with beginning of cycle, they can do it, and *they come here for the very end part or procedure part* . . . Dr. ____ will make a decision that they're ready to be trigged [ready to undergo an egg retrieval procedure], and then they're here for their egg retrieval, their biopsies, their transfers. (IF 7/26/10, emphasis mine)

Since protocols have changed in cases where frozen embryos are transferred at a future time, I assumed that this would make the process more expensive and onerous for cross-border transactions. However, one director explained why the new set of staggered IVF procedures might actually be attractive to patients traveling to the US for sex selection:

There's two options now. You come in for a week, we'll get everything done, you go home. Or, come in for a day, come back in a month for another day. And everybody is choosing to come in for another day. Because remember these [sex selective] PGD patients all have families. . . . And the husband only has to come the first time because the second time is just the embryo transfer. . . . So we're finding this to be tremendously popular with the foreign patients. . . . a lot of the Europeans, a lot of the Asians like the one-day deal. (IF 5/29/15, traveling director, clinic A)

This director also mentioned that the price of a hotel for a full week in an expensive US city adds up, possibly raising the appeal of the "one-day" option.

The global form, then, centers institutionally around the clinic located in largely unregulated legal frameworks. From that node, bi-relational clinic-to-clinic circuits evolve with flows moving between them and across national borders. With the development of satellite clinics and laboratories abroad, the United States also functions as a departure site for providers and patients in cross-border sex selection. Discreet, informal, clinic-to-clinic networks across borders alongside more formal offshore satellite providers make up the global, institutional form of lifestyle sex selection. Within these assemblages, clinics act as endpoints of travel by information, biomaterial, equipment, patients, and providers across borders.

## The US Unbounded

The United States has also served as a departure site in cross-border transactions for sex selection. In general, US-based patients need not circumvent restrictive laws in order to access new sex selection technologies. However, those seeking MicroSort after the trial's termination on US soil and those looking for lower costs might. Providers themselves appear to be active in this area, reaching out to other globally situated and local markets. In this section, I provide a glimpse into the emerging global form of border crossing by providers, first through the particular case of MicroSort/GIVF and then through two other US-based clinical networks that extend PGD services through satellite locations abroad.

When I asked the MicroSort scientific director of the US clinical trial why GIVF began establishing MicroSort overseas prior to a determination by the FDA on its safety and efficacy, he responded:

> The FDA has jurisdiction in the US. It does not have jurisdiction outside the US. So, their involvement in whatever the decision was to go overseas, they were not involved in that. Here's the thing that you've got to realize. The company has been involved in this clinical trial for fifteen years, and conducting a clinical trial, and bringing a medical device to market is first not an inexpensive undertaking, and second it's not being performed for the sake of science. Any company that is developing drugs or devices is doing that with a commercial view in mind. So, identifying international locations where MicroSort might set something up is logical, wouldn't you say? Companies don't spend millions and millions of dollars developing things for fun. (IF 12/8/10–12/22/10)

By pursuing MicroSort as a commercial enterprise outside the United States, GIVF preemptively skirted the FDA's authority. From the establishment of the first lab outside the US in 2009 until the end of the US clinical trial in 2012, GIVF produced two concurrent institutional faces of MicroSort, an investigational device in a US FDA clinical trial and a commercialized product for sale outside the United States. GIVF even authored two websites on MicroSort, one with information on the US clinical trial (www .microsort.net) and one with information about commercially available MicroSort abroad (www. microsort.com). Available in English and Spanish, the internationally focused commercial website offered Skype communication services and a currency converter using "live midmarket rates" to provide up-to-date calculations in other currencies of the MicroSort cost of 13,500 pesos in Mexico or 1,400 euros in Cyprus. In spring 2012, the trial site homepage announced a decision by GIVF's board of directors to terminate the trial and provide a discount on PGD to remaining MicroSort trial enrollees. The trial site has since been taken down and now redirects to the commercial site. In this way, the clinic both complied with and circumvented US state regulatory mechanisms by strategically situating MicroSort labs in spaces where sex selection is not illegal.

One GIVF employee whose primary task related to MicroSort is to look for opportunities to establish laboratories abroad described the process.

He estimated that 80 percent of the time ART clinicians approach GIVF with an interest in providing sorted sperm, and they do not understand the complexity of setting up and running a MicroSort lab. The rest of the time, GIVF seeks out potential locations for labs based on where they get the most requests. Before even addressing issues of feasibility and cost, the interested clinic does the work to understand regulatory issues, which can take several months or even years, and permissibility will rest on an interpretation of laws that often do not have specific language on sex selection. As long as professional ART provision guidelines that discourage the practice are nonbinding and laws remain unspecific, there is an open "not illegal" space for pursuing sperm sorting via MicroSort. Launching into the history of the Greco-Turkish conflict in Cyprus, an embryologist who worked there described to me how the country's quasi-independent political status makes it a favorable location for cross-border reproductive tourism.

> So they have three nationalities, but they have no legal government. They depend on Turkey for everything. There's no law in many, many areas of life. So in reproduction, there is no law. You can do whatever you want. They do surrogacy. They do egg donation. They do everything, sex selection. Now, Cyprus receives a lot, like a lot of medical tourism, in general, for fertility. Their local cases of IVF are almost nonexistent because their population is very, very low. I think like sixty thousand people in the whole country. So it's very low, but there are like seven or eight IVF clinics. All of them receive foreigners. (IF 5/29/15)

Locations that meet the "not illegal" criterion tend to operate discreetly and primarily by word of mouth. For example, while both a lab technician in Mexico and the director of international development for MicroSort confirmed the opening of a MicroSort lab in Kuala Lumpur, Malaysia, in the beginning of 2015, the MicroSort website a year and half later still did not list Malaysia among its lab locations (IF 5/28/15, IF 6/22/15).

It could take six months to a year to purchase and ship the equipment, ensure it clears customs, set it up, and train local technicians to run the lab to standards set by MicroSort (IF 6/22/15). According to a lab technician in Mexico, it took three months after obtaining the facility to receive shipped equipment, test the equipment, and get the laboratory fully certified so it could run its first sort (IF 10/22/2010). A laboratory supervisor does occasionally travel to the facility in Mexico from the United States, but day-to-day contact is made via cameras that allow facility owners in the United States both to communicate with locally based technicians and observe the offshore lab:

> We have a supervisor from the US who comes and checks the lab, and we usually have them on call. If we have a question or anything, we call, and contact with them, and they will answer right away. We're always in communication, but basically, here they only come and visit every now and then, just to review that everything is fine. We have cameras, so they can check the room, so in case we have questions, and they have to see what we're doing . . . We take advantage of technology as much as possible. We don't actually need a person physically here. They can be working over there. They just turn on the camera, and say okay what am I doing here, what should I do here, and they can answer and let us know what we need to do. So, you don't actually need someone here all the time or someone traveling frequently here, because we have technology here. (IF 10/22/10)

Local ART clinics and physicians near these sites willing to provide the technology as part of their product portfolio have become "collaborating" physicians. Because they operate outside of the trial framework and FDA jurisdiction, follow-up, clinical trial data collection, and enrollment criteria such as age restrictions are not enforced. One collaborating physician in Mexico explained the institutional agreement between his clinic and MicroSort:

> With patients coming from abroad [pause], I was trained in the UK, we have the same name, and we have the support of a large clinic in [name of major city on the US East Coast], and they [GIVF] talked to me and we have a lot of experience with patients from abroad, so we have a well-structured method to deal with patients from abroad, and people from MicroSort know this. So, most patients coming from abroad . . . are sent to us. I don't pay them any fee. I don't earn anything by sending them patients for sorting. I don't charge any extra. So, what we have on paper has much more to do with the health department. (IF 11/19/10)

The director underlined the appeal of his clinic's capability of providing GIVF-MicroSort to patients from abroad. He laid out four advantages to Mexico as a global destination site for ART: its geographic and relative cultural proximity to the US and Canada (compared to reproductive tourism sites such as Singapore and Thailand); potential "return reproductive tourism" from a growing second generation of lower-middle-class Mexican Americans who speak Spanish and reside, but cannot afford treatment, in the US; cost; and limited treatment options for women over the age of forty in the US. In the case of this clinical network, both the satellite director and the chief embryologist at the main clinic travel to each other's locations every two to three months to discuss the clinical and laboratory results of their patients. Their sex selective PGD patients tended to come from abroad, while MicroSort with IUI provided a more financially accessible option for local patients (IF 11/24/10).

It appears that GIVF's decision to locate new labs in major Mexican cities was influenced primarily by their potential to serve as cross-border sites for reproduction, rather than to attract local clientele. Indeed, MicroSort does not appear to have advertised much locally. According to one of the lab technicians in Mexico, MicroSort had not launched a major advertising campaign, instead targeting most of its outreach efforts to physicians at conferences and by invitation to an opening event. Among limited promotional materials designed for a local audience, GIVF distributes an informational postcard (see figure 3.1).

One Mexican ART clinic clearly hoped to draw global patient traffic in an advertisement that ran in a medical tourism website:

> Medical tourists seeking to use MicroSort to increase the chances of having a baby of a specific gender should look no further than Mexico City, Mexico. Mexico City, Mexico is the most popular non-beach town in Mexico, and is known for its top fertility specialists. While in Mexico City, Mexico for MicroSort (Gender Selection) enjoy breathtaking sunset views from the Bellini revolving restaurant which overlooks the entire city. (Medstar LLC 2010)

Appearing prior to the end of the US clinical trial on MicroSort, but unburdened by FDA requirements that prohibit making claims regarding the technology's safety profile during investigation, the ad continues: "There

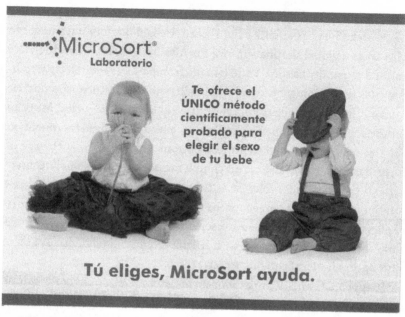

3.1. MicroSort informational postcard designed for local promotion in Mexico

are no reported risks and side effects directly attributed to MicroSort (Gender Selection) in Mexico City, Mexico." The ad then highlights the comparative advantage of cost:

> The cost of MicroSort (Gender Selection) in Mexico City, Mexico is low compared to other countries that provide this service, and easily accessible due to Mexico's healthcare advancements. The average MicroSort lab only charges $1,100.00 per sort.

US-based clinics also construct offshore locations for conducting clinical practice. My research data encompassed one West Coast US-based ART clinic with a satellite arm in Mexico, and one satellite clinic in Mexico connected to an East Coast US-based clinic. I refer to the bundle of clinics connected by ownership across borders as US clinical networks. Both clinical networks in my data provided sex selective PGD in Mexico as well as MicroSort. Without access to PGD screening facilities on site in Mexico, both satellites send cells extracted for PGD testing back to US-based laboratories. Both also have a small number of permanent employees. One staffed two gynecologists, an ultrasound technician, and a hormone specialist, and the other a director and his personal assistant, two nurses, and two embryologists. Within both clinical networks, travel to and from main clinic sites in the United States took place regularly.

The director of the US West Coast clinic explained that he travels about every eight weeks to the Mexican satellite location with a team of embryologists. An embryologist who traveled with him in 2010, when the clinic still had its own in-house lab to conduct PGD via FISH, described the process at that time:

> What we do is we batch patients down there, so we tend to do all the patients in a few days, so it's real intense, 'cause you got to get everything all done within a finite amount of time, 'cause we only have [pause] we do the transfer on day four or five, . . . so we're there for five days so we gotta squeeze all this work in five days. But, pretty much what happens is, same kind of thing, except the slides [on which biopsied cells are placed] we can send out from down there back to the states here. (IF 1/24/11)

The embryologist's reference to batching patients was reiterated by his clinic director. In order to minimize time abroad, a number of women's cycles (the director mentioned forty-seven cases on one visit, and thirty on another) must be synchronized so that the team can perform multiple egg retrieval surgeries on the first day and embryo transfers on the last. He explained, "Because if I go to [name of city in Mexico], I have to get all those forty-seven women to have their eggs ready on the same day, and we do. And, we do it over, and over, and over again" (IF 1/24/11). Clearly designed for the convenience of traveling providers, batching IVF cycles may jeopardize an individual patient's cycle outcome due to suboptimal timing of oocyte retrieval (before or after maturation of follicles) and embryo transfer (during "out of phase endometrium") (Das et al. 2013, 185–186). When I later had an opportunity to meet the team traveling to their satellite location in Guadalajara, I saw that sex selective ART was so thoroughly integrated that it was difficult to disentangle as a separate or unique practice. The team, consisting only of the clinic director and two embryologists, arrived a day earlier than I did and immediately set to work on three egg retrievals and fertilization to create embryos for three PGD cases. The director spoke fluent Spanish with the local staff of physicians, anesthiologists, and nurses, but the two embryologists did not. Inside a hospital, the clinic had a very small waiting room, an office for the traveling director, and a lab for the two traveling embryologists equipped with three workstations—one for handling sperm and paperwork, another with a microscope for identifying and culturing eggs, and a more complex ICSI microscope in the third station to fertilize eggs and biopsy embryos. They had to walk to another area of the hospital to access clinical rooms for egg retrievals and embryo transfers. The traveling director clarified that his personal work schedule rarely changed since he most often relied on telemedicine to do intake consultations, and regularly texted or phoned staff at two other US-based clinic sites in the network. The staff, including nurses, ultrasound technicians, and other physicians, assisted in managing patient cycles in the director's absence because "there's a two-week lead in to every case. And again, I don't have to babysit the patients for those two weeks. I've got to make all the major decisions, but I don't have to be doing everything" (IF 5/29/15). He discussed the importance of impeccable scheduling and communication and demonstrated a keen awareness of the different time zones of the operations.

> Now, when we schedule—you got to be really good at what you do to be able to do this—because when I get back to [clinic on US West Coast], we're going to do fourteen egg pickups. When I came down here, we did a bunch of egg pickups. When I go to [clinic site on US East Coast], we do a bunch of egg pickups and they're all scheduled to hit when they have to hit. So you've got to be a really good scheduler. And if you are, it works, and if you're not, you can't do this.
>
> So there's a huge amount of communication that goes on all the time. I made five or six phone calls this morning. I made a call to the pharmacy pretty quickly. I've got two or three texts. Again, it's still two hours earlier in [clinic site on US West Coast]. It's now late in [clinic site on US East Coast]. So, it will go on all day.

One of the traveling embryologists described a typical workday. They set up the culture medium the evening prior in preparation for morning egg retrievals. Once the eggs are retrieved in the morning, they bring the tubes into the lab to identify and count the eggs, and place them in an incubator for three to four hours to allow them to stabilize. The morning I arrived, I shuffled back and forth from the clinical room to the lab observing this process. In my fieldnotes I recorded the first egg retrieval that morning from an egg donor for a commissioning couple wanting a boy:

> In preparation [the clinic director] put a condom on an ultrasound probe; the nurse filled the tip of the condom with some kind of gel. There was a metal device he then attached to the probe that would hold the pipette aspirator. He has a pedal to begin aspiration, which made a humming sound. The condoms came in blue and pink packages, and he joked with the nurse that they should use blue, because the patient wanted a boy [in this case the patient was not the anesthetized donor in front of him waiting to have her eggs retrieved, but rather the commissioning couple]. . . . The director showed me how each follicle would collapse after he aspirated the egg(s). The eggs were located at the back of the sack and once they dislodged you could see the sack collapse and a little bit of blood dripped in the tube, so that was a good sign, he said. He filled up five vials. (FN 5/27/15)

An embryologist then takes the vials back to the lab to determine an egg count. Once in the lab, I looked under the microscope after the second egg retrieval, and under the guidance of the embryologist, searched for the bluish egg cells, correctly counting eleven. In the meantime, the other embryologist prepped sperm for the ICSI fertilization procedures later in the day. After three to four hours, the embryologists would clean and check the eggs for maturity before ICSI procedures. Once the eggs are fertilized, they return them to the incubator for sixteen to eighteen hours. The next morning they would do biopsies on embryos created a day earlier. Given that these embryologists can handle biopsies for about three cases a day, and each case has on average eight to ten embryos to biopsy, procedural design and capacity remain limited to minimal rather than mass use.

Unlike the clinic director, who traveled regularly between three sites, the two embryologists traveled only between two clinic locations, yet they also felt that their workdays remained basically the same across these sites other than a higher level of intensity in Mexico due to the batching of cases. Their director, who claimed that his clientele coming to Mexico from the US had increased threefold since he began advertising the site as an affordable location for all IVF services two years prior, discussed the possibility of expanding the capacity of the satellite in the future.

Thus, in cross-border sex selection, the United States is situated as both a destination and a departure site within a growing spectrum of traveling practices. The "transnationalization" of clinics (Ikemoto 2009)—the establishment of offshore labs and sites of clinical operations owned and operated by US clinics—has extended these practices into other globally significant hubs. The system tends to escape national and even weaker international regulatory mechanisms. International agency directives that inscribe sex selection as an international issue of concern do not seem to be aware of this emerging global form of sex selection. Cross-border sex selection is not only a global form but also an institutional means to decenter state authority. In this sense, cross-border sex selection constitutes lifestyle sex selection at the same time as it situates such practices within transnational circuits of travel.

## Global Disjuncture:
## International Response to Sex Selection

International agency statements that define sex selection as an international issue of concern address nation-states rather than clinics. They thereby bypass the locus of institutional power in contemporary sex selective ART, along with a growing globalized institutional structure of fertility clinics networked across national borders. Furthermore, although the most recent interagency statement released by the United Nations mentions PGD and sperm sorting, it excludes political, economic, social, and cultural elements related to lifestyle sex selection in its framing of sex selection as an issue of international concern. In this way, the geo-/biopolitical Western site in which lifestyle sex selection developed gets sketched out of definitions of sex selection as an international issue.[5]

The first mention of sex selection in an international document came at the 1994 International Conference on Population and Development (ICPD) in the preformative stages of lifestyle sex selection. Those who drafted and signed the ICPD Programme of Action in 1994 would likely not yet have encountered MicroSort or PGD in relation to sex selection. In chapter 4, the practice of "prenatal sex selection" is interpreted as a symptom of gender discrimination, and (nation-state) governments are urged to act by implementing measures to prevent "prenatal sex selection" (UNFPA 1995, paragraph 4.23). The Beijing Declaration and Platform of Action from the Fourth World Conference on Women made a similar plea, urging governments to "enact and enforce legislation against the perpetrators of practices and acts of violence against women, such as . . . prenatal sex selection" (UN Women 1996, Article 124 [i]).

In 2011, five UN agencies (OHCHR, UNFPA, UNICEF, UN Women, and WHO) released an interagency statement that defines sex selection as a symptom of discrimination against girls and women, reminding governments that they must address the issue as part of their obligation to uphold the human rights of girls and women without compromising on the obligation to provide women with access to safe abortion. The fifteen-page document highlights the problem of sex selection contributing to sex ratio at birth imbalances that exist or have existed in South, East, and Central Asian countries, but warns against stringent legal prohibitions of sex selective abortion that might compromise women's access to needed reproductive health technologies and services (WHO 2011).

The title of the new interagency UN statement released by WHO, *Preventing Gender-Biased Sex Selection*, seems to recognize implicitly the possibility of a non-"gender-biased" form of sex selection. The qualification departs from the 1994 ICPD recommendation, which simply asks governments to prevent (comprehensively) prenatal sex selection. The cover image of three brown-skinned children clad in South Asian garments visually distances itself from the mainstream subject represented on US fertility clinic websites. The document interprets "sex selection in favour of boys" as a "symptom of . . . injustices against women" (4). It thus problematizes the choice itself rather than the act of choosing. A brief mention of "family balancing" in the executive summary treats it as an exception. "Sex selection is sometimes used for family balancing purposes but far more typically occurs because of a systematic preference for boys" (v). Specifically mentioning China, India, Vietnam, Korea, Armenia, Azerbaijan, and Georgia, the document completely leaves out Western regions of the world. Indeed, the latest UN document, focused as it is on the obligations of nation-states, is irrelevant to an institutional system that works to maintain an absence of state intervention, concentrating power in ART clinic institutions. The UN interagency statement exists in an entirely separate internationalized frame that does not implicate the ART clinics driving lifestyle practice. From its inception within the long established contours of UN discussion on population and development to its growing relevance across five UN agencies, the internationalization of sex selection addresses mainly non-Western countries, son preference, and population sex ratio imbalances. Its refusal to incorporate issues related to lifestyle sex selection further accentuates stratification by deepening a divergence between forms of sex selection that are internationally problematized and those whose global form remain mystified as Western and local. In this way, ethical discussions make a number of false assumptions. They assume that sex selection based on son preference is always unrelated to family balancing, when, in fact, most, non-Western families going for a boy do so only after they have had one or more female children (Almond and Edlund 2008; WHO 2011). They assume that majority communities will dilute the potential harms experienced within minority communities (such as sex ratio imbalance), and therefore egalitarian principles ought not trump libertarian ones (Wilkinson and Garrard 2013, 30). They assume that individual desires for a particular sex in offspring can be divorced from culture in one context, but not in another; thus they foreground Western women's individual decision making and deny agency for other(ed) women. Ethical questions that exclusively focus on sex selective abortion abroad, such as those reflected in the UN interagency report, evade the global dimensions of both sex selective ART and abortion.

At the same time, the evolving ethical statements on sex selection made by two formative bodies dealing with ART—the ASRM Ethics Committee (2015) and the ESHRE Task Force on Ethics and Law (Dondorp et al. 2013)—do important institutional work by expanding the ethical gray zones relative to the normalization of sex selective ART. They increase the decision-making power of clinics to determine the ethics of sex selection via ART vis-à-vis the nation-states in which they reside. The ESHRE statement, for example, affirms MicroSort after the uncelebrated end of clinical trial in the US without an FDA approval as "the only proven technology for preconception sex selection"; imagines a "responsible" approach to preconception sex selection via sperm sorting restricted to family balancing; calls for a more expansive definition of medical uses of sex selection; and acknowledges that situations in which nonmedical sex selection is added on to a medically indicated use of PGD "may or may not be against the letter of the law" even where bans on the practice exist

(Dondorp et al. 2013, 6). The ESHRE statement even refers to the "categorical prohibition of sex selection for non-medical reasons as adopted in many Western countries" as "largely symbolic" and to some ethicists potentially restrictive of reproductive liberty (Dondorp et al. 2013, 5). As with the 2015 statement by the ASRM Ethics Committee, the lack of a consensus itself contributes to the migration of professional bioethics toward expanding the ethical gray zones that increasingly normalize sex selective ART. As I suggested in chapter 2, ESHRE and ASRM recommendations do institutional work by reinforcing a status quo that discourages government interference while promoting practice guidelines that increase the interpretive flexibility for clinics deciding how to situate themselves in the global market for sex selective ART.

Government agencies, professional associations, NGOs, and international organizations should question the balanced family as an ideal and family balancing as a rational practice necessarily devoid of bias. Sex selection by whatever means—even when the practices aim to make babies rather than prevent them—and wherever they take place (West or non-West) occur inside the realms of culture and power, and thus are implicated in various kinds of local and global stratifications. International policy recommendations that primarily raise concerns about abortion access in relation to sex selection leave the door open for an interpretation of sex selection as a reasonable family limitation—or biopopulationist—strategy. Rather than only identify sex selective abortion as cause for international concern, which reinforces reproductive binaries (despised/valued reproduction, (over)fertility/(in)fertility, sex selective ART/sex selective abortion), such organizations should broaden their scope to consider more fully the various stratifications that occur in and around sex selection, including border-crossing and ART forms.

# 4

# Contesting the Known

An Arc of Activism on Sex Selection
in the United States

THE UNKNOWABLE ACCOUNT—THE PREMISE THAT IT IS NOT POS-
sible or desirable to identify or quantify a reproductive practice—is central
to the neoliberal zeitgeist. At its core is respect for privacy, liberty, and
the rightness of individual choice. Normally, these values are associated
with mainstream reproductive rights (RR), but US-based reproductive justice (RJ) advocates have also come to embrace the unknowable account in
their work on sex selection in order to protect marginalized and racially
stigmatized groups. In this chapter I trace the activism on the issue of sex
selection as it has evolved since the early 2000s. I analyze how activist
assertions made on sex selection mobilize science to back a set of competing versions of the truth. To this end I reflect on knowability through data
collection and representation of sex selective ART and abortion practices
as well as the power of the unknown. In contrast to sex selective abortion,
the relative permissibility of ART and the fact that the process involves a
positive sex selection, that is, for sexed embryos or sperm carried out by
specialists working in a laboratory, would appear to enable data collection
on its prevalence. Yet, there are a number of sociotechnical factors that
delimit this possibility. In the following section, I discuss the state of data
collection on sex selective ART before turning to campaigns whose truth
claims about sex selective abortion and ART variously refuse data-driven
accounts or reinterpret data.

## Data Collection on Sex Selective ART

In the case of sperm sorting with MicroSort under the conditions of the US trial, GIVF enforced selection criteria for enrolled subjects and kept careful records to meet FDA regulatory standards. Today, we know, for example, that there was a predominance of X-sorts (70.2 percent) for "family balancing."[1] The scientists overseeing the trial speculate that a greater cultural preference for girls or the greater purity ranges achieved for X-sorts might explain this disparity (Karabinus et al. 2014, 10). Author Hanna Rosin drew on this data in her provocative *Atlantic* article announcing "the end of men," and news media attention on sex selective ART in the early to mid-2000s focused almost exclusively on MicroSort data and narrative case stories with images of white American heterosexual couples desiring girls (2010). Since the trial's sponsor, GIVF, withdrew its pre-market application for FDA approval in 2012, information about MicroSort has reverted to proprietary status. Further, GIVF began to sell the method overseas to sites not owned by them, making central compilation of data impossible to impose; data thus becomes unknowable (IF 6/22/15).

As with MicroSort, the very design of PGD technology—particularly the mode of analysis used to study the chromosomes of an embryo's extracted cell and the need of an embryologist to select the chosen embryos for transfer—required the purposive request for sex selection to a provider. In theory, these conditions provide the technical mechanism to quantify requests for sex identification of embryos. Yet, there are many reasons why such numbers remain elusive.

In general, the US has imposed minimal federal regulations on ART practice. The 1992 Fertility Clinic Success Rate and Certification Act remains the single legislative mechanism prompting the central collection of data. For providers with a stake in PGD's continued use, there is little incentive to invite scrutiny through the collection and publication of data. The Centers for Disease Control and Prevention, via the Society for Assisted Reproductive Technology, began collecting data on PGD in 2004, but that data does not break down into reasons for use. We know, for example, that between 2005 and 2014, PGD use hovered between 4 and 6 percent of all IVF cycles (CDC 2016). We also know that a handful of clinics have a proportion of IVF cycles utilizing PGD far greater. For example, the proportion of IVF cycles conducted with PGD at the two US-based clinics featured in my study were 86 and 62 percent, respectively, in 2014 (CDC 2016, Stapleton 2015). An important early survey that did collect data specifically on sex selective PGD was conducted in 2005 by the Genetics and Public Policy Center. It found that 42 percent of clinics offered PGD for nonmedical, sex selective reasons. Of these, 47 percent put no limits on the practice; 41 percent refused requests for first-order births; and 7 percent offered the option only if their patients were already undergoing PGD for medical reasons (Baruch et al. 2008, 1056). Yet, in the absence of ongoing data collection from multiple clinics (other than what the CDC provides), there exist only snapshots of information provided by individual clinics. A 2007 article from the scientific journal *Human Reproduction*, for example, published the sex preferences of ninety-two couples who underwent PGD (a few in conjunction with MicroSort) at the Center for Human Reproduction (New York City) between January 2004 and December 2006. Of those ninety-two, thirty-six selected for girls and fifty-six for boys—hardly evidence for a predominance of "Americans wanting girls." The study concluded, "Gender selection choices were to a statistically significant degree dependent on the couple's ethnicity ($P < 0.001$) . . . there was obvious gender bias in favor of male selection among Chinese, Arab/Muslim, and Asian-Indian couples. In contrast, Caucasian/Hispanic couples demonstrated obvious bias toward female selection" (Gleicher and Barad 2007, 3039).

In addition to the lack of political will to collect data on a broader national basis in the US, the multipurpose design of PGD complicates such a pursuit. Sex determination of embryos is one of the most basic applications of PGD, but its inherently expandable form, in terms of the list of conditions and characteristics for which it can screen, means that sex selection patients can "cross over" to other simultaneous applications of PGD for aneuploidy screening or genetic diagnosis, and vice versa. As one clinic director explained,

> Once you offer the ability to look at the genetics of an embryo, we don't just say we can do boy or girl, we have to sort of let them know everything that we can do and we can do quite a bit, and so as we go through those dialogues with them. They'll say, "Well gosh, it would be good to know this also," and we don't argue with them. We do Down Syndrome,

Patau, Edwards, a lot of the most common heritable aneuploid genetic diseases along with gender selection at the patient's request. (IF 8/24/10)

Later at this clinic, I observed this "crossover" phenomenon close up. Listening in on an initial phone consultation with an African American patient with two girls seeking twin boys, the director offered the patient sickle cell screening after learning that both she and one of her daughters were carriers of the disease. Though the patient did not explicitly request on paper a sickle cell screening and presented herself to the clinic for sex selection, the director offered the PGD sickle cell screening "add-on," which the patient accepted, thereby *crossing over* from a nonmedical to a medical application of PGD.

PGD also embeds within general fertility services as an accessory technology, either to improve IVF success rates (a highly contested claim) or for sex selection. A nurse recounted situations in which infertility patients cross over to sex selection when offered a simple and relatively inexpensive form of PGD testing (via 2-probe FISH):

> We offer the testing, and so they're like, "Why not pay the $2,400 and find out what the sex of the embryos are . . . before we put them in, so if we come back and have a second kid and we already put back a female and we have males frozen, we can come back and choose the sex. . . ." We give them an option. We tell everything that we offer, so that they don't come back and say, "Well, we didn't know we could do that, you didn't tell us." (IF 7/26/10)

In such cases, sex selective PGD becomes an adjunct to a medically indicated infertility treatment. Thus, the line between nonmedical and medical applications of PGD blurs in practice, making it difficult to separate uses of PGD for nonmedical sex selection from other medically indicated uses of the technology.

Around 2009, the mode of cell analysis changed in a way that further complicates efforts to detect and quantify sex selective PGD. Whereas the former method, FISH (fluorescence in situ hybridization), involved screening select pairs of chromosomes, the new method, micro-array CGH, screens all twenty-three pairs of chromosomes. Sex identification of embryos now arrives as a nugget of data alongside other information about the embryo, whether one requests it specifically or not. As one embryologist explained,

> The micro-array stuff—you always know what the sex is going to be because they [the reference lab] give you the XY or XX, whatever it's going to be, we know. . . . They have all that information together, so when we get a report back from [the genetic lab] it'll have the embryos that are safe, the ones that are carriers, and the ones that have the disorder, but each one of those would be either a boy or a girl, so we would know that. (IF 1/24/11)

Since micro-array CGH automatically provides information about the sex of embryos in any instantiation of PGD, it eliminates the requirement of foregrounding an intention to sex select. Rather than having to make an active decision to request a sex determination test, anyone going through IVF may be sold on PGD as a way of ensuring that only "healthy" embryos are put back. With information about sex automatically available, the practice can more easily become a routinized aspect of IVF or merely a matter of information disclosure.

## Campaigning on the Issue of Sex Selection in the US

All these issues aside, the campaign that began in the US around 2001 to raise concerns about sex selection has a checkered history with data— on whether to demand it and how to represent it. Similar to the earlier campaigns in India, advertisements, particularly those targeted at the South Asian community and news media announcing MicroSort and PGD, prompted initial action. What follows is a history of that campaign through my reflection as a participant between 2001 and 2005 and thereafter as observer and through interviews with key activists. I track some of the successes and struggles, particularly around the need to know about sex selection practices and questions that relate to a demand for more or less data and regulation.

My entrée into the issue of sex selection took place in India in the mid-1990s, when I interned briefly as a student and activist at the organization Forum for Women's Health (FFWH) in Mumbai. The history of engagement by FFWH activists in Forum against Sex Determination and

Sex Preselection since its establishment in 1984 in India strongly affected my own feminist framing of the issue. I read documents stemming from the decade-old campaign and listened to firsthand accounts and campaign experiences. Like them, I came to view sex selection as a form of violence against women and girls and a misuse of prenatal diagnostic technologies. In a fact sheet on sex selection that I coauthored for distribution at "Aarohan 2003," a national conference of South Asian organizations and community members in the US dedicated to ending violence against women, we described sex selection as a form of gender-based violence unethically promoted by a profit-seeking industry, a framing not unlike those that had appeared in India two decades earlier among feminists who pioneered campaigns against sex selection (Bhatia et al. 2003). My own organization, the Committee on Women, Population, and the Environment (CWPE), like the FFWH, shared a feminist perspective critical of population control, and we had engaged in campaigns to raise concerns about unethical testing and coercive promotion of contraception. We had challenged the idea that all new contraceptive and sterilization technologies were inherently liberating and brought attention to their potential for abuse in contexts of population control. We were critical of arguments offered by some doctors in India that viewed sex selection as a means to reduce population growth, and aware of advancements in human genetic engineering that might allow sex selection to serve as a stepping stone to expanded consumer options for trait selection. Thus, when in the early fall of 2001 I first learned of the pre-pregnancy technologies and targeted advertising to South Asian communities in the US, we were ready to act.

My first encounter with the issue of sex selection in the US came when two articles on sex selection appeared around the same time in the *New York Times*: "Clinics' Pitch to Indian Émigrés" (August 15, 2001) and "Fertility Ethics Authority Approves Sex Selection" (September 28, 2001). The first piece covered the targeting of sex selection advertisements to South Asian communities in newspapers such as the North American editions of *India Abroad* and *Indian Express*. The second announced the approval of sex selection via PGD by the ASRM Ethics Committee. As explained in chapter 3, the latter article referred to comments made by the acting chair of that committee, John A. Robertson, who misrepresented his committee's consensus position. Yet, this would not be publicly clarified until several months later. In the meantime, I was moved to create an ad hoc coalition to protest the ASRM's purported ethical approval of sex selective PGD. CWPE joined with a newly formed organization, the Center for Genetics and Society, in Oakland, California, in addition to the well-known Boston Women's Health Book Collective (today Our Bodies, Ourselves), Andolan–Organizing South Asian Workers, and Manavi Inc., which works on domestic violence in the South Asian American community. We drafted an open letter signed by over ninety organizations and individuals to the executive director of the ASRM, copied to each member of the ASRM Ethics Committee. It expressed concern over the "actual repercussions" of John A. Robertson's "widely publicized letter," which had mistakenly interpreted the ASRM opinion on PGD for sex selection as ethical approval. The open letter provided the following example.

> According to media reports, [Robertson's] letter is already being used by some fertility specialists to justify offering IVF/PGD even to fertile couples for the sole purpose of sex identification and selection. One fertility center's website seems to suggest that ASRM approves of this practice, citing ASRM's "official opinion" that PGD is no longer "considered an experimental procedure" and then stating a few sentences later that "PGD also lends itself to non-medically indicated gender selection." (Committee on Women, Population, and the Environment 2002)

We further urged the ASRM "to take the earliest and strongest possible actions" to discourage sex selection for nonmedical reasons. Like feminists in India, we made a claim on the appropriate use of a technology, asking that professionals account for and prevent potential "misuses" of new technologies. In other words, we did not seek an outright ban on PGD, but requested that professionals limit their use to "the prevention of serious medical conditions."

Until this point sex selection had not proffered a platform for action in the US, and I remember feeling uncertain about the response to our solicitation of support from internationally known reproductive rights advocates. The action gave us some initial information on how to approach coalition work with mainstream Western feminists on the issue. Some of us thought that the appearance of the new technologies might enable feminists in the West who had shied away from the issue of sex selective abortions to finally clarify their position on sex selection generally. We solicited a position on this issue at a meeting of feminist scholar/activists on new reproductive and genetic technologies in 2004 in New York City. There sixty-five participants agreed to oppose "practices and social conditions that pressure people to select children based on their traits, or to select traits for their children," and also to oppose "sex and disability deselection, but with the important proviso that we could not support laws that would make selective abortion illegal."

By 2005 we were calling ourselves the "campaign against sex selection." Hereafter, I trace the history of this campaign as it went through several iterations with different organizations taking the lead, some dropping out or folding altogether, and new organizations coming into the mix. "Against sex selection" would quickly become a liability in the context of anti-abortion activism on the issue, and organizations would refer to program work in this area as simply "sex selection" or "race and sex selective abortion bans." Therefore, I will use a broad reference, simply "the campaign," to denote work to consistently raise concerns about sex selection from a feminist, RJ perspective of relevance to Asian Americans and others. I refer to "the campaign" in the singular in order to underline a connected thread of activism over time even when there occurred major shifts in its goals and strategies due to changing political contexts and configurations of organizational coalitions and activists who would carry the work forward.

In 2005 the campaign had a new coalition partner, the National Asian Pacific American Women's Forum (NAPAWF). Through both conference calls and face-to-face meetings CGS, CWPE, NAPAWF, and Manavi Inc. brainstormed a three-year strategic plan for our campaign, including activities at regional, national, and international levels. In hindsight, it is clear that we strove to impact how the issue unfolded in the US, but had to grapple with many new dimensions as we took stock of an institutional world of assisted reproductive technologies with which some of us (including myself) were not familiar. We had to delve more into the new technologies without losing sight of the old ones. We had to rethink how to frame a critique as we confronted a range of new and unfamiliar discourses emerging with the practice. We kept a watchful eye out for sex selection ads, blogs, and news media, which we circulated among ourselves. For their overreliance on limited cultural explanations, we resisted frameworks that relied on son preference as the only moral compass by which to evaluate the appropriateness of sex selection technologies. For example, we strategized on how we might make funders such as USAID and the Futures Group accountable for promoting two-child norm policies in India that we knew drove demand for sex selection. We were intensely aware of how our response and actions in the US might impact feminist advocacy against sex selection abroad, and we sought transnational collaboration on the issue.

With regard to issues of data collection and federal government regulation, we debated the importance of drawing a clear line between medical and social uses of the technology and saw a need to collaborate with disability rights communities on these questions. We also discussed a strategy to license ART clinics and limit their use of new reproductive and genetic technologies to specific medically justifiable cases. We saw a need for better data on how these technologies were being used and promoted, and waited in anticipation of a publication by Sunita Puri, a research fellow at the University of California, San Francisco, who we knew had interviewed South Asian women undergoing sex selection about the pressures they faced to have sons. In the meantime, we solicited Puri's involvement in the campaign, co-presenting with her at a few conferences. Operating in an apparent separate sphere from abortion, we did not perceive a demand for greater federal oversight of ART as an overt threat to abortion's legal status. Nonetheless, as an alternative, we contemplated a stance we perceived as less contentious, which would minimally prohibit the marketing of sex selection.

Later that decade core priorities of the campaign began to change as a result of major shifts in the political context and among the organizations that continued the work. Of the four organizations that were still involved in 2005 (Manavi Inc., CWPE, NAPAWF, and the CGS), only NAPAWF has remained centrally involved on the issue of sex selection. For a while after 2005, the Center for Genetics and Society led work in this area until it spun off a new organization in 2008 called Generations Ahead, which then took the helm of organizing on sex selection in the campaign. On the activist scene from 2008 to 2011, Generations Ahead spearheaded a number of initiatives and led the transition into a new phase of changed priorities. Earlier demands for increased regulation of ART were dropped, and in the process the ways in which data was solicited, used, and interpreted also changed drastically.

## 2008—The Tables Turn

In 2008, the same year that Generations Ahead formed, two events prompted changes in the feminist response to sex selection in the US. First, an influential study by Douglas Almond and Lena Edlund published in the *Proceedings of the National Academy of Sciences* divulged sex ratio imbalances at birth among Asian Americans (Korean, Chinese, and Asian Indian). The authors showed that the proportion of boys to girls starts out even among first births within these subgroups, but that it jumps incrementally at second, third, and higher order births if no sons are born. The authors state explicitly, "We interpret the found deviation in favor of sons to be evidence of sex selection, most likely at the prenatal stage" (Almond and Edlund 2008, 5681). Second, US representative Trent Franks introduced a federal bill, the "Susan B. Anthony and Frederick Douglass Prenatal Discrimination Act," to "protect" the fetus from discrimination based on sex or race (bill drafters claimed that abortion providers in the US target black communities, leading to disproportionately high rates of abortion they call genocide). Thus, the very year a reputable study arrived with data that might reveal sex selection as an important issue impacting particular communities in the US, anti-abortion organizations began to mobilize to propose sex selection bans. These bans are embedded within a larger anti-abortion strategy that has sought to circumscribe the right to abortion at the state level ever since a 1992 US Supreme Court decision (*Planned Parenthood v. Casey*) upheld *Roe v. Wade* but afforded states more authority in regulating abortion. The number and types of legislation aimed at restricting abortion have burgeoned at the state level. They include mandating (inaccurate) counseling on the health impacts of abortion, the imposition of mandatory waiting periods, parental or spousal consent laws, and more recent "TRAP" (Targeted Restrictions of Abortion Providers) legislation that requires providers to have hospital admitting privileges and clinics to have ambulatory surgical facilities or to be located a prescribed distance away from schools.

In 2008, Steven Mosher, president of the anti-abortion organization Population Research Institute, proposed banning sex selective abortions as a goal of the "pro-life movement," and Americans United for Life subsequently published a guide to assist state legislators in developing such policy (Kalantry 2015, 146). Between 2009 and 2014, twenty-seven states and the federal government considered sex selective abortion bans and six states enacted such laws. Where the measure did not pass, proponents continued to reintroduce the bill, sometimes year after year (Kalantry 2015; Chou and Jorawar 2015; Jesudason and Baruch n.d.). Law scholar Sital Kalantry describes a common narrative to these proposals: that son preference in China and India has led to widespread practices of sex selective abortion, that Asian immigrants import these cultural practices when they come to the United States, and that bans are needed as a means to prevent sex discrimination and to promote equality (142–143). For proof, anti-abortion legislators drew on the Almond and Edlund study and two further studies by Jason Abrevaya and James Egan et al. that came to similar findings shortly thereafter using different sources of data (Almond and Edlund 2008, Abrevaya 2009, Egan et al. 2011). Sunita Puri's study, which we had long anticipated, finally arrived in 2011 and was quickly also taken up and referenced by conservative, anti-abortion legislators in their bid to ban sex selective abortions. Based on in-depth interviews of sixty-five Indian American women (some of whom used sex selective ART), the study revealed that some faced threats of losing their immigration status or abandonment by their in-laws or husband if they did not produce sons, and some faced physical violence and neglect when sex determination of their fetuses turned out to be female (Puri et al. 2011).

In the face of such anti-abortion mobilization on sex selection, Generations Ahead and other organizations were concerned about compromising abortion access through their advocacy on sex selection; campaign goals and strategies needed to be revised. The need to distinguish feminist advocacy on sex selection from anti-abortion voices became very clear when an aide from Congressman Trent Franks's office telephoned Manavi Inc. and NAPAWF in 2008 with a bid to work together (IF 7/30/15, NAPAWF 2015). Feminist groups recoiled and began to change course.

In the fall of 2008, for example, Generations Ahead, along with NAPAWF and Sistersong, another US-based women of color reproductive justice group, sent a letter to all congressional offices alerting them to the falseness of the gender and racial equality claims made by Trent Franks's Susan B. Anthony and Frederick Douglass Prenatal Discrimination Act.

Generations Ahead then spearheaded the creation of a working group of eighty members with secure access to a website designed to provide information and assist groups around the country fighting anti-abortion, sex selective abortion bans. They assisted local advocacy efforts such as those led by Sistersong and SPARK Reproductive Justice Now in Georgia to defeat a state version of the bill (Jesudason and Baruch n.d., 10).

In spring 2009, Generations Ahead also organized a strategy session and values clarification workshop with the leadership of RR organizations in Washington, DC, and New York City. While it was not difficult for attendees at these sessions to agree on a political strategy to defeat anti-abortion bans on sex selection, they voiced confusion on how they felt about sex selection(IF 10/18/10–10/19/10). In order to assist groups that had been either silent or ambivalent on the issue, Generations Ahead, Asian Communities for Reproductive Justice, and NAPAWF created and released a toolkit in December 2009 under the title *Taking a Stand: Tools for Action on Sex Selection.* Complete with popular education exercises, background, and policy information, the toolkit stressed the importance of protecting abortion rights while not losing sight of significant gender equality concerns related to the practice of sex selection, "including sex discrimination, sexual stereotypes and gender binary assumptions" (Generations Ahead et al. 2009, 6; IF 10/18/10–10/19/10; IF 10/19/10). Generations Ahead continued to stress this dual strategy. As Sujatha Jesudason and Susannah Baruch explained in a project document, "We have worked hard to demonstrate that we can protect women's reproductive autonomy while acknowledging that sex selection is antithetical to women's rights and health. It is possible to work to discourage sex-selective practices while defending women's reproductive decision-making" (Jesudason and Baruch n.d., 10–11). The toolkit refers to sex ratio disparities as "strong evidence" of the occurrence of sex selection, referencing both the Almond and Edlund and Abrevaya studies suggesting the likelihood of such practices among Asian Americans. Similarly, Generations Ahead cited these studies in a letter to the FDA to request greater transparency on the information that would inform their decision on whether to approve MicroSort. Dated November 10, 2009, just when the agency's decision on MicroSort appeared to be imminent, the letter requested a public advisory committee meeting on the sperm-sorting method so that the FDA might hear from non-expert communities potentially affected by the technology.

We urge the FDA to gather input from a range of experts and stake-holders about the potential impact of such products on the public health. MicroSort is currently available only to married couples and only to avoid sex-linked disease and for "family balancing;" however, recent research suggests that in the United States, "family balancing" is having a direct impact on sex ratios in some communities. [Here, the letter footnotes both the Almond and Edlund and Abrevaya studies]. A public advisory committee meeting would allow the FDA to consider its role in addressing these issues, and provide public notice of the FDA's plans for data collection, marketing and labeling requirements.

In this case, the sex ratio data is offered as evidence of a potential negative public health outcome. Advocates from the campaign underlined in interview how they did not want to intervene in FDA decision making with what might be seen as an ideological or political agenda, as had occurred under the Bush administration with emergency contraception. They carefully avoided a stance that might be perceived as a request that the FDA not approve MicroSort. Rather, they viewed their letter as a move for greater public accountability in the process of considering new technologies for the market. Nonetheless, some mainstream reproductive rights organizations, such as the Center for Reproductive Rights and Planned Parenthood, did not sign on to the letter (IF 10/18/10–10/19/10).

It was at this point that goals from earlier years in the campaign, such as improved centralized data collection and central government regulation of ART, began to more fully unravel. The regulatory worlds of ART and abortion seemed to grow closer, or at least their co-implication became increasingly clear. When in 2010 the FDA denied "continued access" to MicroSort for "family balancing" on the grounds that MicroSort did not fulfill a compelling public health need, GIVF tried but failed to convince the FDA that MicroSort could prevent repeat abortions, which compromise women's health (follow-up personal communication with scientific director of US MicroSort trial, June 27, 2011). In response to this move, one advocate from the campaign first indicated to me the benefit of no data. She surmised that GIVF could not reasonably demonstrate to the FDA that MicroSort prevented sex selective abortions if there were no data to document their prevalence in the first place (IF 10/18/10–10/19/10). Thus the lack of data on sex selective abortions appeared to prevent continued access to sex selective ART (specifically MicroSort) for nonmedical "family balancing" reasons in the US.

Furthermore, the legislative strategy to ban sex selective abortion would begin to draw on the very same "evidence"—the Almond and Edlund, Abrevaya, and Puri studies—to make their disingenuous gender equality case against sex selection. The use of sex ratio disparities as a means to demonstrate social harm of sex selection became a double-edged sword. Eventually, the gender equality concerns voiced in the toolkit prepared by Generations Ahead, NAPAWF, and ACRJ in 2009 would diminish in relation to growing racial equality concerns prompted by anti-abortion rhetoric spewing stereotypes of Asian Americans as culturally backward and sexist. After Generations Ahead folded in 2012, NAPAWF began to lead the next iteration of the campaign in an effort to gather different kinds of data that would counter or discredit the claims made by Almond and Edlund, Abrevaya, and Puri.

Clearly, the campaign that had sought to address sex selection from a feminist, reproductive justice perspective had to respond to a changing political context, rethinking several goals and strategies that had predominated in the early 2000s. For example, in relation to an earlier desire for expanded centralized data collection, one advocate began to voice serious reservations:

> Say the CDC starts collecting data about sex selection—the clinics that are doing it, what techniques they are using and what purpose they are doing it for. What would be the purpose of that information both from a progressive perspective and a conservative perspective? An anti-abortion perspective would be about punishing women who do this or who choose to do it. (IF 10/18/10–10/19/10)

Another advocate echoed this concern:

> Data collection might be an area for a better understanding of the practices of sex selection . . . , but we also recognize that's difficult data to get. And data collection in the reproductive health context has often been an anti-abortion tool, and intimidation tool. And so we're really trying to be very careful about where we step. (IF 10/19/10)

Seeing concrete advantages to the self-regulatory model of ART already in place in the US, advocates also revisited a prior goal—seeking greater federal government regulation of ART to prevent what we had previously perceived as illegitimate, nonmedical uses of these technologies. One advocate pointed to the potential danger for women in greater governmental regulation of ART:

> For us it's a stretch beyond just the issue of sex selection. So, we think about how to protect women's reproductive autonomy particularly in a climate where those rights are *so* under attack. Everything and anything is used as an excuse to regulate women and undermine women. And, the women who are going to be the most impacted are poor women and women of color. In that kind of political environment, for now, *for now* the best strategy is professional self-regulation. Frankly, I would much rather have a network of doctors making these ethical decisions than the men in the US Congress. (IF 10/18/10–10/19/10)

Another advocate discussed how advocates themselves might engage in oversight in forms other than government regulation.

> In the context of the US, as a reproductive justice organization it's very tricky. While we've certainly heard other organizations say they think there should be regulation in this area, there haven't been specific suggestions offered that I would be comfortable with. We see the voluntary work with providers, work with patients directly, work with the communities that are most affected by sex selection as the better approach. That's oversight in a different sense. Not government regulation but it is trying to establish some oversight of the practice. (IF 10/19/10)

Thus, to the extent that the campaign remained focused on sex selective ART, the approach turned to helping ART providers adhere to professional guidelines already in place. To that end, they organized an interactive session at the ASRM and published advice in a professional journal to assist providers working with patients considering sex selection.

One further core element of the earlier campaign—the desire to forge transnational collaboration on sex selection—also diminished at this turn.

The political retreat from efforts to forge transnational coalitions occurred, ironically, just as cross-border practices that defy nationally bound regulatory contexts began to increase. One advocate described the "radically different" domestic US context, including abortion politics and healthcare structures, as particular deterrents to transnational work.

> Given the way that Asians—Chinese and Indians—are so stigmatized by [sex selection], [transnational advocacy] actually does a disservice . . . the standard becomes as long as we are not as bad as them in terms of sex ratio disparities and overt son preference, then [sex selection here is] okay, so the transnational comparison becomes a yardstick without really understanding the dynamics. I think about the Chinese and Indian context and how much they are framed by population control policy. . . . I don't think Americans ever understand the nuance, complexity, and history of other advocacy efforts, and so the transnational piece of it becomes to me very devoid of real women. (IF 10/18/10–10/19/10)

This reflection points to the challenges of working across borders on similar issues, especially when a still transnationally potent population control narrative successfully reduces real women and their experiences to a preoccupation with numbers, in this case via sex ratios. In these ways core facets of the campaign in the early 2000s changed fundamentally: from a desire for improved data collection to an understanding of the power of no data; from a desire for government regulation to prevent the misuse of new technologies to a growing appreciation of provider self-regulation; and from a desire for transnational collaboration on shared issues to a focus on domestic contingencies. After 2011, these shifts would continue to deepen as NAPAWF took the mantle of leadership.

In a move that would steer campaign work in new directions, NAPAWF joined two academically tied organizations, Advancing New Standards in Reproductive Health (ANSIRH) and the International Human Rights Clinic at the University of Chicago Law School. In the fall of 2013, the collaborators began to conduct research that could authoritatively discredit claims made by anti-abortion proponents when legislating to ban sex selective abortions. The resulting report, "Replacing Myths with Facts: Sex Selective Abortion Laws in the United States," was released in June 2014.

It questioned whether sex selective abortions are even a problem in the United States, presenting new quantitative analysis and interpretations of the influential Almond and Edlund study. Asserting that "there is, in fact, no way to determine what method has been used to achieve sex selection or whether sex selection has occurred at all based solely on sex ratios at birth," the report invalidates the authenticity of skewed sex ratios as a measure of sex selective abortions (Kalantry 2014, 27). One collaborator said that her "personal big take-away" from the project was to learn that "this notion of sex ratios is extremely problematic and it's not actually a useful way to have the conversation at all" (IF 7/24/15). The report complicates the presumed connection between sex ratios and sex selection by revealing, for example, that Liechtenstein and Armenia, with "predominantly white populations," have more heavily male-biased sex ratios than India and China (Kilantry 2014, 8). Here and elsewhere the report reiterates that the basis of the argument for sex selection abortion bans lies in racial stereotyping, rather than in purported gender equality concerns.

Using more recent data, economists who worked on the "Replacing Myths" project applied and expanded methods used by Almond and Edlund. What they found did not contradict Almond and Edlund, but they emphasized that Asian subgroups contribute more girls than do whites to the total population if all births are taken into account. "When we compare the overall sex ratio at birth of foreign-born Chinese, Indian, and Korean families to the sex ratio at birth of whites born in the United States, we find that these Asian groups have *more* girls on average than whites" (Kalantry 2014, 16). Thus, while the report does not question Almond and Edlund's findings per se, it does question those who have used the study to create a perception that all Asian Americans carry culturally determined sex bias and do not value girls. It highlights that studies used to corroborate claims made in legislative proposals to ban sex selective abortions (Almond and Edlund 2008, Egan et al. 2011, Abrevaya 2009) all have limitations. Some use old data or fail to provide a comparative analysis with other racial groups. The "Replacing Myths" report cautions that findings from the single qualitative study (Sunita Puri et al.) referenced in legislative proposals to ban sex selective abortion are not representative of "South Asian women" because the study relied on interviews of "only 65 women" (2014, 20). As a co-participant with Puri for a short time in the earlier years of this campaign, I admit that the report's apparent dismissal of this work as simply not representative gave me pause to reflect on the radical political shifts the campaign had undergone.

Other strategies the report uses to combat racial stereotyping are to question whether son preference will necessarily manifest through sex selection practices and reappear wherever Asians migrate. Emphasizing the difference that a changed geopolitical context makes, the report contrasts socioeconomic factors between India and the US. It suggests that greater access to pension systems and the absence of a patrilocal family system (where married couples live with the husband's parents) are factors that could decrease demand for sex selection. Unlike earlier campaign literature, the report does not forthrightly take a stand on sex selection. Only in the very last sentence do the writers admit, "We do not support the practice of sex selection by any means, but rather than combating discrimination, sex-selective abortion bans perpetuate it" (28). Less than five years earlier, the campaign primarily framed the issue as a concern with the gender discriminatory impact of sex selection that could not be resolved with restrictions on abortion. "Replacing Myths" redirected the primary concern to the racial discriminatory impact of sex selective abortion bans. The campaign would soon take a more offensive approach to combating what NAPAWF called "wolves in sheep's clothing," referring to disingenuous use by anti-abortion legislators of civil and women's rights language to defend their proposed bans (NAPAWF 2013).

In 2013 the American Civil Liberties Union filed a lawsuit against the state of Arizona on behalf of NAPAWF and the National Association for the Advancement of Colored People (NAACP) of Maricopa County in Arizona asserting that the sex and race abortion ban passed there in 2011 violated "the Equal Protection Clause of the 14th Amendment because it targets and stigmatizes Black and AAPI women" (NAPAWF 2015). Although unsuccessful (the case was dismissed first by a district court in Arizona, and upon appeal, also by a circuit court in California), the action provided collaborators with the opportunity to assemble more academically backed evidence on the harmful impact of such laws. Social psychologists, constitutional scholars, advocates for Asian immigrant rights and black women's health all filed amici curiae in support of the plaintiffs. They compiled sophisticated evidence, citing a burgeoning area of research that relates stereotyping and stigma to physical and psychological health problems. They placed the Arizona law within a historical context of legislation targeting and discriminating against Asian Americans in the United States based on a perception of (rather than actual) threat (NAPAWF 2015). Finally, the campaign successfully sought resolutions by city councils with large Asian immigrant populations such as those in Oakland and San Francisco, California, to denounce sex selective abortion bans as racially discriminatory and bad for women's health.

In the last fifteen years the campaign has followed an arc that has led it to a very different place. The goals and strategies of the campaign have undergone dramatic change in response to a shifting context; one current campaign representative could barely recognize some of the recommendations made in "Sex Selection: A Fact Sheet," dated 2005, written and archived by her own organization. In particular, the advocate regarded strategies of "stopping the advertising," to "persuade clinics not to offer," and "to develop regulation and oversight policies for" sex selection technologies and practices as no longer applicable (NAPAWF 2005, IF 7/30/15). Indeed, campaign representatives deemphasized the importance of sex selection as a stand-alone issue apart from more broadly framed concerns around gender norms and son preference. As one veteran activist put it, "If I were to do a campaign now, I would do a much more expansive one, like, 'Let's talk about gender norms in our community and how they show up in terms of violence and how they show up in terms of sex selection and how they turn up in terms of LGBT issues.' I wouldn't lead with sex selection as the issue" (IF 7/24/15). I now turn to an exploration of the significance of changes in the US-based sex selection campaign for reproductive justice and the politics of knowledge production and use.

## The Struggle for Reproductive Justice and the Politics of Knowledge Production and Use

Conceptualized by women of color activists in the US, *reproductive justice* takes as its central concern the consistently devalued reproduction of disadvantaged groups. Advocates focus on the right to have and raise children in supporting environments just as much as the right not to have them. Broad-based by definition, RJ movements in the US account for multiple and intersecting oppressions faced by disadvantaged groups (Silliman et al. 2004, Luna and Luker 2013). Thus, RJ claims foreground notions of justice based on the social and political recognition of particular subgroups within a population, the "other," which sociologists Luna and Luker specifically define as "often poor people, people of color, people with disabilities, and people with non-normative gender expression and sexualities" (345). Feminist philosopher Nancy Fraser defines misrecognition of subgroups as an impediment to social justice through their "status subordination" or "institutionalized patterns of cultural value [that] constitute some actors as inferior, excluded, wholly other or simply invisible, hence as less than full partners in social interaction" (Fraser 2001, 24). In their elaboration on reproductive justice, Asian Communities for Reproductive Justice (ACRJ) exemplify this idea.

> The Reproductive Justice framework is rooted in the recognition of the histories of reproductive oppression and abuse in all communities, and in the case of ACRJ, in the histories of Asian communities and other communities of color. This framework uses a model grounded in organizing women and girls to change structural power inequalities. The central theme of the Reproductive Justice framework is a focus on the control and exploitation of women's bodies, sexuality and reproduction as an effective strategy of controlling women and communities, particularly those of color. Controlling a woman's body controls her life, her options and her potential. Historically and currently, a woman's lack of power and self-determination is mediated through the multiple oppressions of race, class, gender, sexuality, ability, age and immigration status. Thus, controlling individual women becomes a strategic pathway to regulating entire communities. (ACRJ 2005, 2)

In distinguishing reproductive *justice* from a service delivery model of reproductive *health*, and a legal and advocacy model of reproductive *rights* focused solely on the individual, ACRJ insisted that all three are equally necessary to "achieve the goal of ending reproductive oppression." Yet in practice, reproductive *justice* movements developed in critique of a reproductive *rights* mainstream movement, which had exclusively focused on individual liberty.

In order to protect abortion rights, increasingly under threat during the 1980s' conservative backlash under Reagan, pro-choice activists within organizations such as the National Abortion and Reproductive Rights Action League and Planned Parenthood made a strategic decision to attract potential libertarian supporters to protect the legality of abortion by narrowing the frame of reproductive rights to its legal justification in privacy (Silliman et al. 2004, 32). The achievement of legalized abortion in the US came in the Supreme Court's *Roe v. Wade* (1973) decision as a negative right of government non-interference in order to protect the privacy of individuals. Yet, the apparent universality of such a right was easily contradicted through a political reality for some groups of women, for example, poor women on public assistance, who had neither privacy nor the means to enact it. On the heels of abortion's legalization in the US, the passage of the Hyde Amendment assured that no federal monies could be used to finance abortion procedures for low-income women relying on publicly funded health-care coverage (Silliman et al. 2004, Luna and Luker 2013). Increasingly alienated within the mainstream movement for reproductive rights, women of color developed perspectives that focused on the ways in which anti-abortion strategies increasingly combine with broader political-economic policies to compromise not only access to safe and legal abortion, but also the sustainability and well-being of marginalized communities (ACRJ 2005). Luna and Luker capture this tension: "Although rights are a part of justice, the nominal universalism of rights, especially the right to privacy, masks structural disparities based on race, sexuality, gender, class and disability, among other axes" (2013, 343). The political ethos of reproductive justice as it developed in the US in the late twentieth century challenged a reproductive rights framework that had become libertarian, abortion-centric, and focused on market-driven notions of choice.

As already mentioned, my own activism in the early 2000s on sex selection was affiliated with a feminist critique of population control—a grounding stake of reproductive justice movements. Fifteen years thereafter the issue of sex selection still situates within a framework of reproductive justice, but now on different grounds: the criminalization of abortion. Redirected away from international population control and the profit-seeking fertility market, campaign activists have focused on a different enemy—anti-abortion groups. Another pillar of reproductive justice activism, the criminalization of reproduction has been meticulously documented by scholars affiliated with an advocacy group called the National Advocates for Pregnant Women. Since the 1990s, the cases in which women's pregnancies were a critical factor in legal claims that led to their arrest, detention, or having to face forced medical intervention has risen sharply (Paltrow and Flavin 2013). This occurred concurrent with a rapid rise in rates of incarceration. Predictably, low-income and minority women, predominantly African American, have faced the brunt of the increased policing and criminalization of pregnant women—most often for charges of illegal drug use while pregnant. While Asian Americans have not figured prominently among these cases, the politics of sex selective abortion bans easily ignites within the public imagination the idea of Asian women having a criminal predilection to endanger or kill their children, especially girls.

The criminalization of reproduction in the US also rests on a set of feticide laws. Thirty-eight US states have feticide laws, all of which arose in response to violence against women with the express purpose of protecting pregnant women. They impose additional penalties against violators by accounting for fetuses as separate and additional victims. In 2004, a federal version called the Unborn Victims of Violence Act was passed (Paltrow and Flavin 2013, Paltrow 2015). Although states have invoked feticide laws minimally, reproductive justice advocates feared that states could use such laws to penalize pregnant women for their conduct during pregnancy or for seeking an abortion. Paltrow and Flavin argue, "Even when women are not charged directly under feticide laws, such laws are used to support the argument that generally worded murder statutes, child endangerment laws, drug delivery laws, and other laws should be interpreted to permit the arrest and prosecution of pregnant women in relationship to the embryos or fetuses they carry" (2013, 323). They also recognized that a very thin line separates criminalizing pregnant women from recriminalizing abortion. The latter came to pass in spring of 2015 when the first conviction of a woman for the crime of feticide occurred in the US to an Indian American woman named Purvi Patel. While Patel's case did not involve the allegation of a sex selective abortion, the simultaneity of Indiana's senate support for a sex selective abortion ban and the conviction of a South Asian American woman there for feticide appear not entirely coincidental. Indeed, the only other woman, Bei Bei Shuai, charged with feticide in Indiana was also of Asian (Chinese) origin. This suggests increased salience in US political culture of a visual and figurative discourse associating Asian women with criminalized reproduction, particularly feticide. That laws governing feticide might implicate the very women they were intended to protect seems uniquely tied to US abortion politics and culture, yet feminist groups in India have faced a similar danger. They struggle to prevent reinterpretations of the Indian law banning sex selection that may endanger the right to access abortions.

In retrospect, several feminist scholars and activists in India involved in campaigns during the 1980s to oppose sex selection, which culminated in a federal law banning techniques of sex determination at the prenatal and preconception stage, questioned early messages and visuals that could be interpreted as anti-abortion (Ravindra 1993, Gupte 2003). Feminist scholar Nivedita Menon articulated an early critique of Forum against Sex Determination and Sex Preselection's legalistic strategy, fearing it might impinge on India's liberal abortion law even when the campaign took pains to avoid reform to the Medical Termination of Pregnancy Act (Menon 1995). As the issue has mainstreamed, celebrities and prominent government officials, rather than feminists, have kept the issue of sex selection in the forefront of public attention in India, but often in ways that endanger the right to access a safe and legal abortion. Feminist activists have had to maintain pressure on the state not to interpret the Preconception and Prenatal Diagnostic Techniques Act in a way that would compromise abortion access. In 2011, for example, feminist activists sent a letter of protest with 250 signatories to the Speaker of the Maharashtra Legislative Assembly objecting to suggestions made within the chamber to treat "female foeticide" as murder (Varghese 2011). In light of these transnational parallels, I provide here a brief interpretation of the Patel case in order to explain the shifts in context that have led to a re-anchoring of reproductive justice claims made by activist communities in relation to sex selection in the US.

In the summer of 2013, Purvi Patel visited a hospital in South Bend, Indiana, in need of care. The doctors, recognizing the signs of a recently terminated pregnancy, suspected Patel of wrongdoing, and called the police. What followed was a series of attempts to locate the fetus and interrogate Patel. Arrested for two apparently contradictory felony charges against her—that she conducted an illegal abortion and that she neglected her live baby, Patel was tried and convicted of both in early 2015 and sentenced to twenty years in prison (Bazelon 2015, Kaplan 2015). With the strong backing of reproductive justice advocates and pro bono legal representation, Patel later successfully appealed the feticide charge and was freed in September 2016 after her child neglect sentence was reduced (Revesz 2016).

Patel's case crossed the line of applying feticide laws to criminalize rather than to protect women's conduct around their own pregnancies. Indiana prosecutors explicitly invoked the state's feticide law to prosecute Patel for an illegal abortion. According to the state of Indiana's code on criminal law and procedure, "A person who knowingly or intentionally terminates a human pregnancy with an intention other than to produce a live birth or to remove a dead fetus commits feticide, a level 3 felony," which does not apply to legal abortions (Indiana Code 35-42-1-6). Whether or not the expelled fetus had lived became a point of contention in court. Several news articles focused on the reliance by the prosecution on an antiquated and scientifically debunked method to prove that it had taken a breath (Bazelon 2015, Kaplan 2015, Diaz-Tello 2015). A fetus that died in utero might have supported the claim of miscarriage, but would not absolve Patel from the charge that she conducted an illegal abortion (i.e., feticide), for which the state sentenced her to six years in prison. A live fetus not only implicated her for feticide but also secured the claim of child neglect, for which she was sentenced to twenty years (Gandy 2015). Either way, the state ensured that Patel would face a paradoxical situation in which the only way out of the courtroom was through the doors to prison. The state's supposed interest in protecting life (of the fetus) exposes itself as a political strategy to induce what the feminist philosopher Judith Butler calls precarity—a "condition in which *certain populations* suffer from failing social and economic networks of support and become differentially exposed to injury, violence, and death" (Butler 2009, 25, emphasis mine). From the moment Patel walked into the hospital to save her own life, she became an enemy of the state and her life became precarious, conditioned on the loss of liberty. Such precarity applies to "certain populations," and it did not take long for Asian American and immigrant rights organizations such as NAPAWF, South Asian Americans Leading Together (SAALT), and Apna Ghar to recognize the significance of Patel's identity as an Indian American woman as highly significant to the outcome and meanings of the case. In addition to their leadership to oppose sex selective abortion bans, NAPAWF spearheaded an online advocacy movement, #freepurvipatel. Although separate, both of these campaigns mutually implicate one another as they occupy the same cornerstone of reproductive justice advocacy related to the criminalization of reproduction.

Highly visible in public images, Patel's racialized and gendered body activated several narratives related to devalued reproducers such as "unfit mothers" and "baby killers." Such narratives increasingly overlap as they surround the Patel case. Although they originate in the separate policy contexts of the US and India, their effects breach those jurisdictional borders within the diaspora. For example, the population control narrative has a long history of implicating Asian women as reproducing excessively, beyond their capacity to care for their children. According to Malthusian logic, an inability to control sexuality and fertility implicitly became a means to question the parenting ability of women within high-fertility contexts—to condemn their reproduction as irrational and beyond their capacity to care for their children. Gender and development scholar Kalpana Wilson argues, "Not only is population control by definition concerned with regulating sexual and reproductive activities, but, like earlier colonial projects of enumeration and measurement, is marked by an overwhelming preoccupation with racialized notions of 'deviant' sexuality'" (Wilson 2012, 85–86). In her reading of Malthus's famous essay on population from 1798, Carole McCann analyzes his naturalized descriptions of the "promiscuity and bad mothering" of women from India—tied, of course, to the lack of "sexual civility" in Indian men. These "knowledge products" of Malthusianism endure (McCann 2009, 152, 144). Indeed, observers of the trial emphasized that Patel's "demeanor and affect" were "put on the stand" in ways that appeared to "prove" her deviance (Diaz-Tello 2015). The fact that she did not cry during the proceedings seemed to implicate her as uncaring even before her conviction. At sentencing, Judge Elizabeth Hurley's reprimand that Patel "treated the child literally as a piece of trash," oft repeated and circulated in the press in connection with Patel's image, almost too easily awakened a connection between brown women and neglectful, irresponsible mothers in the public's mind.

In addition, the trope of savage baby killer continues to have narrative force in relation to Asian women's bodies in the US. Although Patel was not being prosecuted for murder, the lawyer representing the state of Indiana (appellee) during Patel's appeal, heard on May 23, 2016, narrated a story of her killing a baby rather than terminating a pregnancy.

> May it please the court. When she was 25 weeks pregnant with a viable
> fetus and acting outside the parameters of legal abortion the defendant

self-administered powerful drugs to prematurely terminate her pregnancy intending that her unborn child die. When he was instead born alive, the defendant made no attempt to provide him with the medical care necessary to preserve his life but instead insured his death by cutting the umbilical cord without clamping it, putting him in the trash, and lying about his existence. (http://content.ilight.net/supremecourt /05232016_0200pm.mp3; 26:45)

Judges hearing the appeal took several minutes of questioning to unpack this opening in order to clarify that Patel had, in fact, not been charged with murder, and that no evidence existed to suggest that she knew the fetus was alive at the time she disposed of it. Added to the usual anti-abortion narrative devices used here, such as referring to the fetus as "unborn child," is a consistent gendering through the use of "he" as pronoun. Although ART is apparently a less embattled reproductive technology than abortion, the relative acceptability of gendering a fetus via sex selective ART may be interpreted alongside feticide laws as conferring personhood (and then potentially also victimhood) to the fetus. Activist literature by Generations Ahead, NAPAWF, and others consistently balk at the assertion of "prenatal non-discrimination" by supporters of selective abortion bans. They do so by pointing out their slim to nonexistent track records fighting discrimination on the basis of sex, race, and disability but also by questioning the curious lack of equal concern among supporters of the bans for sex selective ART.

Although unstated, racial stereotypes give the attorney's story narrative force. The process by which Patel's behaviors transform into criminal ones depends on deeply embedded cultural notions that associate certain subgroups within the population with criminality. These include vestiges of a colonial narrative of a "savage baby killer," which recalls a racially "othered" subject. In her discussion of the Patel case, WGS scholar Ashwini Tambe recalls a moment in her classroom when religious moral codes constructing Asians as savage baby killers clouded her students' ability to grasp the multiple dynamics of power implicated in sex selection practices:

When I taught the topic of global reproductive justice several years ago at Georgetown University, a flagship Catholic institution, I frequently noticed that many of my students became especially animated when we turned our attention to China and India. . . . many students already knew about the problem of female feticide and infanticide in these countries; it was clear to me that for those who had been raised within strong Catholic anti-reproductive rights environments, China and India were widely maligned. These countries were understood as places with a *criminal predilection for sacrificing life.* The very real and pernicious social problems of misogyny and son preference compounded by economic inequality in China and India, all of which local activists have struggled against, had been displaced by accounts that equated national identities with these national crimes. (Tambe 2015, emphasis mine)

In a postcolonial era in which high rates of sex selective abortions are associated with the global non-West, anti-abortion advocacy easily resurrects the "savage baby killer" narrative. Tambe's students could quickly recognize the problem of sex selection but only in terms of a reductive formation of "othered" national identity that was simultaneously racialized and criminalized. A second gendered narrative related to sex selection centers on the "sex-starved, violence-prone" surplus men of the non-West, who will form a "mobile army" that "will threaten China's sociopolitical stability and perhaps make it more bellicose abroad" (Greenhalgh 2012, 137). Similarly racialized, this narrative began to circulate in the Western scholarly fields of demography, public health, and security studies by the mid-2000s. It highlights how Western perceptions of sex selection practices in Asia are tied to nativist, conservative fears of immigration as infiltration by ethnically marked men who are prone to violence.

Sex selection joins female circumcision, bride burnings, and veiling within feminist theory's growing list of culturally challenging topics prone to relativistic responses when imagined outside the West or libertarian ones when inside. The US-based campaign on sex selection began to shift in ways that increasingly looked libertarian as well, even while it oriented firmly within the activist arena of reproductive justice. One advocate highlighted for me the dilemma that ultimately pivoted campaign goals: "So do you want people to oppose sex selection because they think of it in terms of racial stereotypes? I'm not sure that's a good outcome" (IF 7/24/15). For these reasons, the evolution of the campaign provides a distinct optic through which to grapple with the interdependence of reproductive autonomy and justice anew. Drawing on both theorizations of reproductive justice and feminist science and technology studies perspectives on knowledge production and use, I explore the transnational "dislocation" of sex selection as an issue in the United States.

Years before the Patel case, the tactical strategy deployed by the campaign retooled to focus energy on countering legislative proposals to ban sex selective abortions. They did so in the name of reproductive justice. The fear that such bans might lead to racial profiling and added scrutiny of Asian women's decisions and actions around reproduction became real when Asian American advocacy organizations realized that the pernicious stereotypes that undergirded Patel's conviction also motivate the passage of sex selective abortion bans. Thus, NAPAWF and allied organizations uphold unencumbered access to abortion services as a racially just strategy, rather than as a means to uphold the rights of individuals above all else. This is not a case in which the individual trumps the social, or rights trump justice. In spite of the historically contingent rise of reproductive justice as a way to decenter focus on abortion rights advocacy to the exclusion of equally important reproductive issues for marginalized groups, the evolution in the US campaign on sex selection reveals an interesting inversion, where abortion rights advocacy was now pursued for the sake of justice.

Not surprisingly, a number of mainstream reproductive rights organizations have backed the advocacy to oppose sex selective abortion bans. Many of them have duly followed the lead of reproductive justice organizations in crafting positions and strategies of their own on this issue. For example, the Center for Reproductive Rights drafted a position statement included in the appendices of *Taking a Stand: Tools for Action on Sex Selection*, a toolkit prepared by Generations Ahead, NAPAWF, and ACRJ. It outlined four reasons to oppose sex selective abortion bans, highlighting their ineffectiveness in promoting gender equality (Generations Ahead et al., 2009). The Guttmacher Institute website frames the issue similarly to the Chicago International Human Rights Clinic, NAPAWF, and ANSIRH in their document "Replacing Myths" (Kalantry 2014). It acknowledges sex selection as a problem of gender discrimination in East and South Asia that does not necessarily migrate to the United States along with the people who come from those regions. It also suggests that bans stigmatize Asian American communities and put an undue burden on providers, who are required to "second-guess" Asian women's reasons for seeking an abortion (Kalantry 2014, Guttmacher Institute 2016).

Campaign activists account with pride their ability to impact the mainstream reproductive rights response, which moved from hesitancy to articulation of a nuanced position and action (IF 7/24/15, IF 7/30/15). At least on the issue of sex selection, they bridged the advocacy gulf between RR and RJ movements apparently on their own terms. However, given the tendency for an empty adoption of RJ terminology without the accompanying intersectional grit related to reproductive oppression, as well as the increasing pressure on RJ activists to recenter abortion amidst challenges to its legality in the US, it is reasonable to question whether the joint RJ and RR opposition to sex selective abortion bans sacrifices the rigor of justice. How is it essentially different from the mainstream, pro-choice reaction to anti-abortion politics as usual? Through its narrow emphasis on the racial discriminatory impacts of sex selective abortion bans within the US, has this approach weakened its concern for gender and global inequality explicit in the early years of the campaign? To answer these questions, it is helpful to explore the enactment of a reproductive justice response on the issue of sex selective abortion bans through the politics of knowledge production and use.

Feminist science and technology studies (STS) scholar Susan Greenhalgh documents how population sciences construct particular truths, and how the processes that go into the making of statistics become obscured in the assertions of a particular reality. In her review of the process by which China's one-child policy became the only solution to a "crisis" framed by population scientists, Greenhalgh notes: "Chinese population science—like all population sciences—is not detached from, but linked to and in varying degrees shaped by politics. . . . I also contend that the numbers of science tell a truth, but it is only one truth. That is because the numbers are created by particular human beings working in specific historical contexts, and both the people and the context leave their imprints on the science that gets made" (2003, 165). Likewise, the experience and evolution of the feminist campaign on the issue of sex selection in the US demonstrates the functionality of sex ratios in the political assertions made by different constituencies that construct the problem of sex selection in varied ways. In the early 2000s the campaign employed sex ratios as a way to bring attention to the potential social harms of sex selection that fertility markets seemed likely to ignore, but this changed. The campaign now questions the meanings of such numbers, refuting whether a problem related to the devaluation of daughters among Asian families in the US actually exists. For example, NAPAWF executive director Miriam Yeung now dismisses the problem of sex selection. Explaining the issue in a webinar, she stated:

> Race and sex selective abortion bans . . . criminalize doctors for providing abortions based on the race and sex of the fetus. While copying language and heroes of social justice and racial justice movements these bills try to fool us into thinking that these proponents are actually feminists and actually anti-racist champions by so-called preventing the abortions of black babies and Asian female babies. But, we know a wolf in sheep's clothing when we see one. You can't give someone rights by taking away their rights. And this is essentially what this law is about. PRENDAs [Prenatal Nondiscrimination Acts] as we call them were developed by the [indiscernible] movement to chip away at abortion rights for all women. *In this case they do so by exploiting stereotypes of black women and Asian women and they developed a so-called solution for a problem that doesn't even exist in the United States.* (NAPAWF 2015)

This assertion follows two significant moves made in "Replacing Myths." Of the six myths contested, two deal with sex ratios: (1) that "male-biased sex ratios at birth are proof that sex-selective abortions are occurring," refuted because sex selection can take place via ART (rather than abortion) and (2) that empirical studies such as the oft-cited work of Almond and Edlund "prove that sex-selective abortions based on son preference are occurring in the United States" (Kalantry 2014, 6). Instead, the document asserts, Asian subgroups have more girls overall than white Americans. In other words, the authors compare the proportion of girls in absolute numbers of children between Asian and white populations, assuming both groups had the same number of children (15). This move does not refute Almond and Edlund's findings so much as highlight alternative numerical data that has the power to reframe the narrative. The strategic shift puts forth a reproductive justice claim about knowledge use and representation. By questioning the effect of sex ratio data that directs a "so-called" solution to a "problem that doesn't even exist in the United States," Yeung demonstrates that the presentation of sex ratio data constructs a particular reality that has the power to obscure others. Contradicting what is presumed to be known by legislators arguing for a selective abortion ban, Yeung continues:

> While legislators claim that Asian-Americans are aborting their female fetuses because we have son preference, a recent study by the University of Chicago Law School shows that actually Asian-American families are having *more* female babies by proportion than white families. During a legislative hearing for this law in Arizona, Representative Rick Murphy was asked to present data about sex selective abortions in Arizona, and he replied, "We *know* that people from *those* countries and from *those* cultures are moving and immigrating in some reasonable number to the United States and to Arizona, and so with that in mind why in good conscience would we want to wait until the problem does develop and bad things are happening and then react when we could be proactive." (NAPAWF 2015, emphasis in original)

In her emphasis and tone, Yeung mocks Murphy's presumption to know about Asian culture. The specter of Asian immigration raised by Murphy and others arguing in support of sex selective abortion bans led legal scholar Sital Kalantry to question whether the recent spate of sex selective abortion bans is actually an anti-immigration strategy, given that a higher percentage of states that considered or adopted such a law experienced a greater than 70 percent rise in the Asian population in the first decade of this century (2015, 141). Indeed, Kalantry's observation demonstrates how population control strategies might look very different depending on context. Even though they appear diametrically opposed, sex selection *provision* in India and sex selection *bans* in the US both target the reproductive behaviors of subgroups of Asians with respect to dominant global or national populations. As such, they function as boundaries that keep particular groups of people on the periphery. Carole McCann reveals how population statistics functioned as Orientalist devices in mid-twentieth-century demographic theories, and how they can be taken up by any number of projects to draw boundaries between "us" and "others."

> The equation of the aggregate mean with the commonplace individual is the primary fiction of population statistics. These self-portraits meld the aggregate, the typical, and the ideal together in mobile arithmetic

figures that have been a staple of demographic discourse since Thomas Malthus and Lambert Adolphe Quetelet. The continual slippage between the aggregate mean and the average man homogenizes the "us" of a nation (gender, race, etc.) and sharpens "our" contrast to "others." In this way, population statistics can serve any number of fluid and shifting policy debates, population discourses, and political agendas. These debates and agendas shift through time as the solidity and significance of the numbers are taken up by different constituencies pursuing new and renewed projects of their own. (McCann 2009, 145)

Adopting a strategy reminiscent of those often employed in feminist critiques of population control (see UBINIG 1993), Yeung challenges the abstractions created in numerical representations, this time redirected at sex ratios that tell a purported truth about deviant Asian reproduction. While a detailed study of the social and scientific construction of the sex ratio would exceed the scope of this chapter, recent US-based activist unease with sex ratios as representational devices warrants a brief look into their rise on the international stage.

Just as demographers began to register India's declining fertility and population growth rates at the end of the twentieth century, national and international attention shifted to the sex ratio. Prominent demographers like Amartya Sen dismissed the idea that the recent practice of sex selective abortions could have a major impact on already skewed sex ratios (imbalanced sex ratios existed since the origin of census taking in India in the late nineteenth century [Visaria 2007]). It is often forgotten that Sen's famous idea of "missing women," which was written with respect to adults, did not comment on child sex ratios or sex ratios at birth. The piece problematized sex ratio disparities precisely in areas that had experienced recent rapid economic growth and notably did not make any mention of sex selective abortions (Sen 1990). Yet, the simultaneity of new awareness of sex selective abortions practices in the global non-West with the appearance of Sen's influential piece "More Than 100 Million Women Are Missing" led to the convergence of the two in public discourse, with a causal connection increasingly implied if not stated explicitly. In mainstream news media ahead of the 1994 Cairo conference, for example, a 1991 *New York Times* article boldly headlined "Ultrasound Skews India's Birth Ratio" drew on a UNFPA report that similarly suggested that rampant sex selective abortions were driving sex ratio imbalances. "It is generally recognized that adverse sex ratio occurs not because fewer girls are born (or conceived) but because fewer are allowed to be born or to survive" (Gargan 1991, 13). Today, sex ratios and sex selective abortions are so often referenced in conjunction with each other that each acts as a sign for the other. Grappling with the ethics of sex selection in the UK, Wilkinson and Garrard claim in their 2013 report that "one of the main bad consequences that could follow from permitting sex selection is population sex imbalance. . . . In some countries where sex selection is widely practised *it has indeed led to population imbalance*," and reference is made to China, South Korea, and India (Wilkinson and Garrard 2013, 30, emphasis mine). Similarly, in campaign literature that I coauthored in the early 2000s, we also suggested this causal link: "Where its use is most widespread, prenatal diagnosis for sex selection reveals clear discrimination against the girl child, *leading to* severe gender imbalances in the population" (Bhatia et al. 2003, emphasis mine). The 2015 ASRM Ethics Committee statement on sex selection for nonmedical reasons cites an impact on sex ratio among the "social justice concerns" related to the practice: "The recognition that many girls are 'missing' in countries such as China and India *as a result of* infanticide, abortion, and efforts to achieve preconception sex selection is longstanding" (Ethics Committee 2015, 1420). Therefore, implicitly or explicitly, the existence of adverse sex ratios has come to mark and serve as evidence that the practice is widespread.

As UK sociologists and public policy scholars Shahid Perwez, Roger Jeffery, and Patricia Jeffery point out, the idea that sex selective abortions are "the single most important reason for the consistently declining sex ratio" has become "conventional wisdom" (Perwez et al. 2012). Since the co-implication of the two seems rather intuitive, few scholars and policy analysts have questioned this relationship. However, in "a demographic epiphany," Perwez et al. point out the possibility of exaggeration, particularly in the absence of data on families that stop having children if their first and second born are sons. Perwez et al. demonstrate that those practicing sex selection in a region of India did so only after having one or two daughters. The authors suggest, therefore, that the "stopping behavior" (i.e., families that stop having children after one or two boys) may be more responsible for skewed sex ratios than those selecting against girls via abortion because these families contribute on balance more girls to the population (Perwez et al. 2012). In addition to mirroring the claim made in the "Replacing Myths" report, which focuses on Asian subpopulations in the US, this argument underscores how efforts to limit family size are integral to sex ratio disparities.

Several other studies cited in a UN interagency report confirm the importance of birth order to the phenomenon of masculinizing sex ratios at birth: "In general, sex-ratio imbalances across affected countries increase as birth order increases. As a result, the ratio is more skewed among second, third or higher birth-order children compared to first-borns. This indicates an increasing desire for boys as the number of girl children increases" (WHO 2011, 2). Notably, the UN does not refer to these cases as "family balancing." A brief mention of "family balancing" in the executive summary treats it as an exception: "Sex selection is sometimes used for family balancing purposes but far more typically occurs because of a systematic preference for boys" (v). This discursive measure retains *family balancing's* ostensible sex neutrality, which would guard against an application motivated by sex bias. The report interprets "sex selection in favour of boys" as a "symptom of . . . injustices against women" (4). The cover photo of three brown-skinned children clad with South Asian garments alongside sex ratio statistics from East, South, and Central Asian countries constitutes a racialized and nationalized formation of the problem. While it is not my intention to question the validity of the direct correlation between masculinizing sex ratios and sex selection practices motivated by son preference, I argue that the representation of sex ratio as a *knowable* and measurable indicator of a problem that is indelibly tied to racialized and nationalized identities reinforces a hierarchy of nations much as fertility rates did from the middle of the twentieth century onward. Moreover, it is not just that sex ratios today act like fertility rates did in the past, but rather that these figures coalesce in a reinforced population control narrative that continues to represent Asians as irresponsible breeders.

It is not inconsequential that sex selection was taken up on the international stage in Cairo in 1994, within the very venue that had for decades indexed a nation's development status on the basis of fertility and population growth rates. UN fora directly associate national identity with "gender-biased" sex selection in a way that strongly overlaps with the stigma of the population control narrative, which had already rendered non-West women as overly fertile and unfit to manage their own reproduction. The basic rationale behind the decennial population conferences during the twentieth century had been neo-Malthusian—the idea that overpopulation would compromise the efforts of formerly colonized nation-states to modernize and develop. It was a system of nation identification and recognition based on knowable census data—statistical, measureable references, while it also re-hierarchized and neocolonized non-West countries (McCann 2009). The 2011 UN interagency document *Preventing Gender-Biased Sex Selection* (WHO 2011) highlights sex ratios in ways similar to how fertility rates functioned in the past—as markers of backwardness and underdevelopment. Sex selection is defined in this document as a problem of global concern only for those nations where sex ratios are out of balance, specifically China, India, Vietnam, Korea, Armenia, Azerbaijan, and Georgia. The document does not include diaspora or the selection practices of Euro-American groups, adding to the perception that such groups sex select only for presumably unbiased "family balancing" reasons.

I now return to the question of whether the RJ and RR coalitional response to sex selective abortion bans is accountable to multivariate impacts of reproductive oppression. By focusing on the unjust racial stereotyping on which the legislative rationale for sex selective abortion bans in the US depend, does the campaign unravel the carefully crafted dual and intersectional response that has continued to raise gender equality concerns "including sex discrimination, sexual stereotypes and gender binary assumptions" (Generations Ahead et al. 2009, 6; IF 10/18/10–10/19/10)? The problematization of sex selection practices in "Replacing Myths" (Kalantry 2014) occurs only in relation to practices in India and China. The document, as with Yeung's intervention mentioned above, does not question whether culture is implicated in practices of sex selection where they may be considered a problem for gender equality. "Replacing Myths" includes two box inserts, one on India and the other on China, which cast the damning evidence of imbalanced child sex ratios for each country alongside descriptions of religio-cultural elements such as a patrilocal pattern of residence and the Hindu belief that only sons can perform funeral rites in India as well as "deep-rooted Confucian values" and a "dominant patriarchal system" in China that sustain son preference. Markedly absent is any mention of population control with respect to India. However, China's one-child policy *is* additionally implicated as one of the "primary reasons for the increases" in the male to female sex ratio at birth alongside the availability of prenatal diagnostic technology. Yet, without an accompanying feminist critique of international population control, this acknowledgment might actually reinforce US anti-abortion politics. As Greenhalgh explains, an anti-abortion interpretation partly influenced "United States public discourse" on China's one-child policy through media depictions of "coerced abortions, family planning jails, orphanage dying rooms, and much more" that "gave fresh life to Cold War notions of China as 'totalitarian Other,' the foil to the 'democratic West'" (Greenhalgh 2003, 163). Attributing China's imbalanced sex ratios to China's one-child policy without understanding the policy's historical connection and contingency relative to Western population science and policy priorities contributes to the idea of sex selective abortion as an alien, threatening cultural practice.

Accompanied with the acknowledgment of cultural influences in India is a "comparison to the United States" section that highlights differences of context such as the existence of pension systems, the absence of a patrilocal pattern of residence among families, and a decreased significance of dowry. Overall the document does not question the importance of sociocultural factors as drivers of sex selection practice abroad; it questions whether such elements necessarily adhere to their peoples that move into the diaspora. This argument forms a rebuttal to the suggestion that immigrants will inevitably bring the "social evils" they practice with them when they come to the United States. Yet, it participates in the neo-imperial Othering practices that maintain the East as subject to an unchanging culture and the West as more democratic, free, and equal to an extent that may even obliterate or "dilute" rather than compound or complicate unique forms of intersectional gender oppression faced in immigrant communities.

A comparison of the US-based RJ opposition to sex selective abortion bans to two other perspectives developed on sex selection with respect to immigrant community "sub-groups" in the UK (Wilkinson and Garrard 2013) and "minority groups" in the Netherlands (Saharso 2003) assists my inquiry into the justice claim made in the US. For example, professional bioethicists Wilkinson and Garrard argue:

> There are ethnic subgroups in the UK who *do possess the cultural features* which favour the production of an imbalanced population. But this result

won't necessarily affect the majority of people in the UK, since members of such subgroups may choose to have children with other members of the same group. If they do marry outside their sub-group, then these cultural features are likely to be diluted; if they don't do so, then the population imbalance will only occur inside that sub-group. And though that imbalance may well be harmful to the members of that group, that doesn't seem a sufficient reason for constraining the reproductive liberties of all of the rest of the population. (2013, 30, emphasis mine)

Unlike the US-based RJ assertion of autonomy *for the sake of* (racial) justice that opposes sex selective abortion bans, Wilkinson and Garrard present a typical autonomy *over* justice perspective. Sociologist Sawitri Saharso, writing on the issue in the Netherlands, comes to a similar conclusion as Wilkinson and Garrard. Yet her stance, informed by feminist bioethics, acknowledges a tension between the feminist principles of "sexual equality" and "autonomy of women." Since, as she surmises, "sex-selective abortion hardly occurs in the Netherlands," she argues that "amending the abortion law to prevent sex-selective abortion would seriously violate the right of autonomy of *all* women." Saharso concedes, however, that "if we put the autonomy of women first, then we should also accept a woman's possible *culturally inspired desire* for a sex-selective abortion" (Saharso 2003, 210, emphasis mine). She resolves this tension by arguing that sex selective abortions ought to be prevented "by other means" (210). All three perspectives oppose sex selective abortion bans and treat "culture" as an unchanging, fixed characteristic of a group of people that is regrettable but to be tolerated (Wilkinson and Garrard), regrettable but to be addressed by other means (Saharso), or regrettable, but not (necessarily) applicable to contexts outside their places of origin (Kalantry 2014). My concern with this treatment of culture echoes that of anthropologist Miriam Ticktin in her direct response to Saharso. While agreeing with Saharso's overall argument as well as policy recommendations, Ticktin raises provocative questions about Saharso's depiction of "a culturally inspired desire for a sex selective abortion." She asks:

What is this culture that makes women commit [sex selective abortion]? Where are these patriarchal traditions from? The impression given is that they are static, fixed across geography and history, and the difference between India and the Netherlands is simply one of numbers. What is not clear is that other aspects of these women's contexts shape their cultural practices, and that cultural practices are always contested, changing, and often contradictory: minority women's practices are shaped as much by their class backgrounds, their immigration status, their minority status, whether they face discrimination and racism from the majority population, their literacy, and so on. They are influenced by global inequalities and disparities of power. *Focusing on a notion of culture and cultural respect as the main source of contention depoliticizes the question of why these women have become a focal point without significant evidence about [sex selective abortion], ignoring the histories and legacies of colonialism and racism that now shape the imagery around Muslim and "third world" women.* It also ignores the question of power and domination: what are the forces that help shape these women's lives—how do the global inequalities which lead to immigration shape their worlds, practices and choices? Indeed, it has been shown that the racism faced by minorities has often worked to engender practices that distinguish minority from majority, precisely as a form of agency and resistance. Similarly, the rates of violence against women in immigrant communities have been shown to be correlated with powerlessness, racism and economic hardship: here, what immigrant communities hold in common is their structural position, not their supposedly violent or patriarchal cultures. (Ticktin 2005, 267–268, emphasis mine).

Ticktin's critique equally applies to Wilkinson and Garrard's deployment of a limited understanding of "culture," but to its credit, the US-based RJ response does produce a more nuanced understanding of the structural position of Asian Americans. The RJ opposition to sex selective abortion bans in the US asks why women of Asian descent living in the US "have become a focal point without significant evidence about [sex selective abortion]." Yet, their rigorous critique of racism does not apply to contexts outside the US. Their condemnation of sex selection practices in China and India duplicates religio-cultural explanations of son preference apparently relevant only to contexts inside India and China. Such descriptions, I argue, only deepen the very stereotypes they seek to undo. Although the RJ authors of the "Replacing Myths" report in the US rightly contend that context matters, this position allows them to condemn sex selection for its gender discriminatory impacts abroad and not at home. Ticktin challenges us to think precisely about how, rather than simply whether, cultural contexts should matter, especially in relation to multiple and overlapping systems of power and inequality. Women's studies scholar Mary John critiques many studies on sex selection for their "tendency to simply repeat the usual list for son preference in patrilineal and patrilocal societies—as security in old age, for carrying on the family name, for lighting the funeral pyre and so on, compared to an equally generic view of daughters as burden" without needed "denaturalization and historicization" (UN Women 2014, 20–21, 41). John further provides a critical assessment of simplistic "violence against women" and "political-economic" explanations for sex selection when cast in similarly "generic" ways, using "loosely" applied terms such as "gender discrimination and bias" without regard to specificity of context and multiplicity of factors (35–36, 41–42). Susan Greenhalgh provides an equally compelling critique of the use of "patriarchy" in demographic studies of China's sex ratio disparity: "Left undefined and unattached to a robust theory of gender that recognized gender's already classed, raced, and sexed nature, the term patriarchy has done some not so helpful work . . . Failure to carefully define and delimit patriarchy has allowed ugly biases about certain men, certain ethnic groups, and certain classes to enter the field of discourse unchallenged" (2013, 146). Greenhalgh highlights how a lack of an intersectional approach to the study of sex ratios has led rather easily to a racialization of the problem, the consequences of which are manifest in US anti-abortion strategies. However, the same could be equally true in reverse.

The RJ recourse to the power of the unknown to challenge the racist stereotyping utilized in anti-abortion arguments for sex selective abortion bans in the US is understandable. Contesting the racist presumption of knowing what *those* (Asian) cultures bring to the United States is paramount. The position rightfully takes a stand on the misrepresentation of sex ratio data in legislative arguments for sex selective abortion bans. Nonetheless, my concern is that an RJ position that acknowledges sex selection as a problem only in relation to India or China may reproduce simplistic ideas of culture that ignore transnational social, political, and economic as well as transcultural elements at play in enactments of and contestations related to sex selection in the US. Further, the intersectional dimensions of the issue of sex selection might get lost if racial equality concerns supersede those related to gender and global inequality and justice, especially if we dismiss the idea of sex selection as a problem at all. An RJ response that derives from histories of reproductive oppression ought to be wary that unknowability and autonomy, as compelling as they may appear in the quest for racial justice, can work as "master's tools," (Lorde [1979] 2015) that is, they also fulfill the neoliberal, dominant pro-choice paradigm that has historically defended the right to abortion over and above other reproductive justice concerns. In order to hold the RR mainstream more fully to account, rather than risk slipping into a position that does their bidding, RJ movements must complicate their perspective on sex selection practices, whether they occur by ART or abortion, here or abroad. Similar to the RJ interpretation of birth control practices, which views them as potentially liberating or exploiting depending on context and structural dimensions of power at play, we must continue to walk fine lines, in this case between anti-abortion proponents on the one hand, and population control advocates and market forces on the other.

# Conclusion

## Toward a Feminist Intersectional Perspective on Sex Selection

IN A RECENT SPECIAL ISSUE OF *SCIENCE, TECHNOLOGY AND HUMAN Values* devoted to entanglements of science, ethics, and justice, Laura Mamo and Jennifer Fishman argue that few STS scholars explicitly engage with "justice"—either as an object of analysis or as a goal. In response to the comparative lack, they call on STS to reflexively engage with justice, while at the same time noting that in their experience issues of power and politics have been particularly addressed in STS within feminist episte-mology. They highlight a long-standing tension between what they call normative and descriptive/constructivist claims within STS when they ask, "Are the normative dimensions of ethics and justice compatible with constructivist approaches that often drive STS projects? Can we move from using 'ethics' and 'justice' as *objects of analysis* in STS to becoming goals in and of themselves?" (Mamo and Fishman 2013, 7). Ultimately, they insist that "discursive and structural framings are not mutually exclusive" (9), and they call for STS to examine, employ, and work with the concepts of justice and ethics in new ways and with increased specificity. To that end, I have sought in this book to cull and sharpen the interpretive strengths of two main concepts applicable to sex selection—"stratified reproduc-tion" and "reproductive justice"—because the former is valuable for its descriptive power and the latter for its articulation of normative goals.

Originally coined by Shellee Cohen, the term *stratified reproduction* gained prominence through Faye Ginsburg and Rayna Rapp's influential 1995 volume *Conceiving the New World Order*. Ginsburg and Rapp define the term as "power relations by which some categories of people are empowered to nurture and reproduce, while others are disempowered," and "arrangements by which some reproductive futures are valued while others are despised" (Ginsburg and Rapp 1995, 3). That which is stratified or valued differently is the reproduction of different groups of people relative to one another. In an encyclopedic entry on the term, Amy Agigian clarifies that categories of valued and despised reproduction relate to markers of social difference: "Reproduction can be, and is, stratified along multiple axes of social status and exclusion. Relevant inequalities include gender, race, class, nation, sexual orientation, age, health and disability status, and legal status" (Agigian 2007, 4827). Yet, I have argued that a process of pinning markers of status along such axes to reproductive strata—valued or not valued—might reinforce reproductive binaries, allowing interpretations of sex selection that remain blind to intersecting oppressions. Fertility-enhancing technology does not simply correlate with white privilege and valued reproduction. We have seen how a gender-exclusive analysis allows culture to function as a marker of identifying those uncultivated populations whose reproductive practices are gender biased and therefore despicable. Meanwhile, the Western "culture of no culture" is accepted by many as without gender bias, not in need of ethical interrogation, and unfairly having to bear infringements on reproductive liberty on account of uncultivated others in its midst.

I argued in chapters 1 and 2 how a cultural economy of difference, or Orientalism, undergirded the processes that formed lifestyle sex selection. I began with a historical focus on the development of the techniques of MicroSort and PGD as they moved from the experimental realm in the agriculture industry to human medicine and within human medicine from a medical purpose to the *anticipation* of a nonmedical (what I have called lifestyle) application. Significantly, their residence and context in sites of high science and Fertility Inc. came with associative meaning, and their acceptance in the medical realm hinged upon successful disassociation from abortion and, particularly for MicroSort, from preconception methods deemed unscientific. Thereafter I traced their *incorporation* as biomedicalized practices within Fertility Inc. and the "making up" of biopolitical subjectivities that can (rightfully) engage in them, including the family balancer and gender dreamer. These boundary-making developments, which rely on and reinforce Orientalist markers of difference, crucially constituted the lifestyle form and content of sex selection as ethically acceptable via ART.

The Ginsburg and Rapp anthology also addresses stratified reproduction in the context of nationally or culturally bound sites such as abortion in Romania, ARTs in the UK, contraception in Brazil, and prenatal diagnostic screening in Southern California. Such an approach would leave much out of focus today as current activities, especially those related to cross-border reproduction, take place in increasingly enmeshed transnational and biopolitical contexts involving multiple technologies and subjects. Rigid notions of inequality conceptualized via strata may not always apply to shifting and intensifying "global reproscapes," defined by Marcia Inhorn as "circulation of actors, technologies, money, media, ideas, and human gametes, all moving in complicated manners across geographical landscapes" (2011a, 87).

Moreover, activities related to reproduction today have increasingly broadened in a way that does not directly relate to the production or care of offspring. Women engage in many new kinds of activities involving their reproductive bodies that do not necessarily have their own reproduction (or prevention thereof) as their main aim, but rather, a breadth of goals such as their future reproduction, their own economic security (in service of the reproduction of others), a contribution to research, or the fulfillment of parental or family formation identities—the case in point is lifestyle sex selection. Those activities may or may not result in a child, but it is important that feminist theorists of reproduction conceptually capture situated activities that people engage in that involve their reproductive bodies toward multiple ends, not merely to have or to prevent having their own child, but to live particular kinds of lives. Indeed, reproductive technological practices have grown in kind (if not number) so much that the traditional notion of a reproductive right to "decide freely and responsibly the number, spacing and timing" of children, "and to have the information and means to do so," seems almost quaint (Article 7.3, Programme of Action, International Conference on Population and Development, 1994). Even those who engage assisted reproduction in the hopes of having a child understand the odds that they are likely not to get one. Sarah Franklin's (1997) conceptualization of IVF as a "hope technology" captures this idea. To encompass the full meaning of reproductive technological practices, then, a frame of analysis should center the process of engagement with a myriad of technological forms as an end itself, rather than a means to an end. The focus should shift from the reproduction of humans as an end to the varied technoscientific activities or processes that involve reproductive bodies for different ends. Thus, stratified reproduction, as a description of inequality, ought to be understood as a dynamic, intersectional process, rather than a static condition.

As I have already described, *reproductive justice* emerged within the activism of literature attuned to the abuses of population control, which sought to acknowledge reproductive oppression and broaden a narrowly defined framework that had come to center narrowly on the right to abortion. The concept shifts us away from the use of *reproduction* (noun) to *reproductive* (adjective). The term can bring focus to a broader range of inequalities that associate with reproductive bodies and processes as they gain significance in connection to promoting egalitarian principles of social justice for marginalized communities who have faced reproductive oppression. The term has cohered beyond its activist-oriented origins, but remains precarious when its invocation, like a buzzword, proliferates based on various and even competing ideas. Michelle Murphy's historical analysis on the meanings of "health" is instructive here. As she describes,

> Health . . . was reinvigorated in the 1970s as a domain of value that authorized national and transnational interventions. Indeterminate in form, "health" underwrote an array of projects, from community clinics, to environmental regulation, to international development regimes. In other words, the qualities of indeterminacy and extension were productive of intensive investments into health as a domain in which questions ranging from decolonization, to increased GDP, to women's liberation—and not just illness—were at stake. (2012, 51)

Similarly, "justice" through "indeterminacy and extension," and especially when erased of its historical contingency as an idea meant to challenge predominant notions of individual liberty and choice related to reproduction—can be invoked in a way that supports those very same principles. Indeed, McGowan and Sharp bring into sharp focus how "bioethical approaches to sex selection and justice" have variously claimed libertarian or relativist ideas, rather than egalitarian ones (2013, 273–275). As with "knowledge" and "health" or any other "domain of value" (Murphy 2012, 51), "justice" claims require robust situation. Further, claims making for reproductive justice must reach beyond classic issues such as sterilization abuse and coercive contraception, without losing sight of them, in order to intervene in an increasingly complex transnational reproductive economy.

The global assemblage of lifestyle sex selection comprises techniques, sites, people, and regulations. In this book, I have argued that the market viability of lifestyle sex selection depends on a cultural economy of sameness or multiculturalism sustained through new subjectivities such as the global biocitizen and the structural mechanisms of globalization. These include (de)regulatory actions by the American Society for Reproductive Medicine to maintain clinic authority in deciding ethical practice combined with the *extension* of the practice to global markets. I have described the mundane tasks and operations of transnational clinics as well as the importance of regulatory patchworks and growing ethical ambivalence (or gray zones) even where the practice is otherwise condemned and/or illegal. The entire complex of cross-border clinical and laboratory networks falls outside the purview of UN agencies. In raising concern for growing disparities in child sex ratios as well as the actions taken by nation-states to address them, these agencies explicitly refer to "family balancing" as an exception to gender-biased sex selection practices. While they present data demonstrating that families in the non-West undertake sex selection to seek an elusive son after having one or more girls, they maintain an artificial boundary between son preference and family balancing. The transnational operations of clinics and labs function structurally in a way that decenters and diminishes nation-state authority while asserting authoritative governance over reproductive practices.

Finally, by tracing the arc of feminist activism on sex selection in the US through shifting political contexts, I have critically reflected on reproductive justice claims, particularly their *contestation* of what is and is not known or can and cannot be known about sex selection practices. I account for a number of dramatic shifts in this campaign over time: from making the case that sex selection ought to be an issue of concern to the claim that it is not really a problem; from demanding greater clinic accountability to ethical guidelines and centralized data collection to supporting the (de) regulatory status quo and fearing the potential harms of data collection; and from a primary focus on gender to racial subordination.

In conclusion I call for a feminist intersectional perspective and approach that refuses to be captured on either side of reproductive binaries: ARTs/contraceptives, individual/population, (in)fertility/(over) fertility, and pro-natalism/anti-natalism. Such a strategy will promote a more dynamic understanding of stratified reproduction alongside a more robustly situated definition of reproductive justice. The absence of a nuanced feminist perspective on sex selection that is inclusive of varied technologies, alongside an increasingly articulated anti-abortion perspective against sex selective abortion, leaves US feminists with Asian backgrounds limited options to intervene. Mobilized to defend abortion rights in reaction to proposals for sex selective abortion bans, for example, they can be placed in the awkward position of having to defend their right to sex select or even deny their own community's practice of engaging in sex selection. Bridging the ART/abortion divide in the issue of sex selection represents an opportunity and challenge to move beyond a narrow framework of reproductive choice that centers on the right to abortion at the expense of a more inclusive position. The local politics of banning sex selection in China, India, the UK, or Canada tend to spur a transnational market for sex selective ART practices to sites where they are not illegal. Adding to this, the local politics in the US of banning (exclusively) sex selective abortion tends to bolster ART's relative moral status. Can feminists deliver a reproductive justice perspective that condemns, both politically and morally, stratified sex selection? Sex selection has always functioned as a gender-essentializing technology, regardless of particular cultural context or technology of use. Now, within transnational, biopolitical economies and cultures, significantly imbricated by the local politics of abortion, sex selection functions as a technology of racialization as well. At the same time, the biocultural contexts of Fertility Inc. confer class-based, transnational biocitizenship, which can (temporarily) remove or mitigate the strictures of race/ethnicity while reinforcing the strictures of binaried gender and cisnormativity. Only a feminist, intersectional perspective can attend to these growing complexities and shifting inequalities in reproduction.

Without an interpretation on racialized gender, anti-abortion legislators in the US try to boost their moral upper hand by claiming that laws to ban sex selective abortion promote gender equality. The feminist reproductive justice campaigns on sex selection in the US easily recognized this strategy as disingenuous. These campaigns brought sharp attention to the harmful racial stereotypes proliferating in calls to ban sex selective abortion, and their potential to increase surveillance and policing of pregnancy and reproductive decision making targeted at Asian communities in the US. But, I worry that the tendency to frame sex selection as "not an issue" for Asians here (in the United States) even if "back home" (in Asia) the practice justifies limitations on reproductive liberty, can play into the West/non-West divide that reinforces so many forms of stratified reproduction. A robustly situated reproductive justice perspective on sex selection requires that feminists keep an eye out for multiple technologies, sites, people, and regulatory forms in order to account for and address mechanisms of social control and subordination that recur via biomedicalization and biopopulationism.

I have argued that lifestyle sex selection represents a case study of biomedicalization. This case has been fairly easy to make. For the first time humans can seek a medical intervention to address their desire for a sex-specific child. Many facets of biomedicalization apply to lifestyle sex selection, such as "extensions of biomedicine through technoscience" and the focus on enhancements, among others (Clarke et al. 2010, 22–24). While the theorization of biomedicalization explicitly engages Foucauldian notions of biopower and biopolitics (4–6), my specific case makes a further claim. I contend that lifestyle sex selection also represents a current permutation of population control, or what I call biopopulationism. Just as with medicalization, vestiges of an older regime, the international population control order, continue and reconfigure in new ways that no longer require an explicit pathologization of and interventions to control human numbers. Unlike the Foucauldian notion of biopolitics, feminist critiques of population control framed power primarily in negative terms that subordinated targeted groups of people. Vested in the "sovereign" of state institutions, international bodies and philanthrocapitalist entities such as the Rockefeller and Ford Foundations, this power had a "capacity to define who matters and who does not, who is *disposable* and who is not" (Mbembe 2003, 27). As such, the regime of international population control prominent in the latter half of the twentieth century was at once an instantiation of both bio- and necro-power. The project of controlling the fertility of the poor by targeting them for sterilization or long-term contraception played out on gendered and racialized bodies within a global hierarchy made up of modern or backward nation-states.

A growing international women's health movement during the 1980s condemned population control, particularly abuses related to the coercive testing and promotion of fertility-control technologies that routinely overlooked health risks and issues of consent. These feminist politics embraced the issue of sex selection because it was interpreted as an example of the harm to girls and women caused by population control. The issue quickly catapulted from the relatively marginal sites of activism locally to national and international stages. Once "prenatal sex selection" made its way into the concluding document of the ICPD in 1994, it became a stock issue to demonstrate concern for women's empowerment, gender equality and equity, issues at the "heart" of the ICPD (UNFPA 2011). Sex ratios at birth soon became yet another statistical device to rank countries. For example, the World Economic Forum (2015) has since 2006 incorporated sex ratios at birth in calculations of gender gaps by country, purported to have a correlation to a country's economically competitive status.

The timing of this ascendency is important, for it is precisely the ICPD that marks a pivot in the old international population order away from population control to a new framework of reproductive health and rights. Here, biopower neoliberalized, shifting focus from states to markets and from populations to individuals. Feminists first articulated concerns about sex selection as part of an integrated critique of the abuses of population control in the 1980s; the rapid climb of the issue to national and international stages at the ICPD by the mid-1990s included it in the very discursive processes focused on reproductive health and rights that would erase that "population control" frame. That left only "cultural son preference" as the primary motivation and explanation for demand. Population control could no longer be implicated.

Since it was precisely through a feminist critique of population control that I came to the issue of sex selection, perhaps my call to retrieve this aspect of the analysis is both personal and political. Throughout the time of most intense data collection there were a few jarring moments that forced me to self-reflect. A clinic director I shadowed in practice made an off-hand, sarcastic comment about the South Asian couple we had just encountered, who were undergoing PGD for a boy. He said, "They don't look so evil, do they?" I immediately responded, "Of course not!" Did I think they were evil? Did I somehow convey that I thought they were evil? Or, did I just somehow come on the receiving end of his quest to demonstrate the ordinary (multicultural) sameness of his patients? Feminist condemnations of the practice (with which I had identified) never questioned the integrity of any individual woman's decision to pursue sex selection within her situated context. This, however, did not mean that there were no other questions to be asked.

Another moment occurred when I spoke by phone to a self-help website author, a woman who had also undergone PGD for a boy. An initial casual exchange led to my off-the-cuff disclosure that my own children include a girl and a boy. Later in the course of our conversation she insisted, which I did not deny, that I could then not possibly understand the longing she and other women had experienced for a child of specific gender, because I had without striving for it what many of them so dearly wanted: the ideal "complete" and "balanced" family.

How could I reconcile this reading of my family makeup, with my experience being the third daughter in an Indian family without sons? No one hid the fact that my parents planned a third child hoping for a boy. Before sex selective ART, and sex selective abortion, having another child was a form of testing the odds of getting a child of desired gender. Only as an adult have I pondered the moment of my birth, often relayed to me casually. Apparently my parents, who had been well prepared with a boy's name, were so disappointed that I was a girl, they could not name me. It was the well-timed intervention of an aunty friend visiting the hospital who had a name handy: "If not Rajan," she said, referring to the name they had in store, "she will be Rajani." Even though I was never made to feel unwanted, I have begun to look back and wonder at the consequence of my birth, which connected as it was with "tying the knot" (tubal ligation) immediately thereafter, definitively ascribed my family of origin as sonless. Is this partly why my Buas (father's sisters) treated my mother so poorly? Is this why my mother had my hair cut so short while my sisters wore braids and ponytails? Delving into how my own personal experiences and family makeup might affect my views on the issue and motivation to pursue this topic only reveals the connection between the personal and political. Perhaps it is the incomprehensible knowing that I might never have been that drives my search for answers about these practices, especially in all of their cross-cultural, transnational complexity.

Though I attended my first pro-choice march in Washington, DC, in 1989, it was the feminist critique of the politics of population control exposed to me by German and Indian feminists that called me to feminism. The first major text I read in German on Indian population policies and family planning thoroughly undid my taken-for-granted knowledge about India's so-called overpopulation problem as the cause of all its developmental woes (Lambrecht and Mertens 1989). Feminist critiques of population control brought me and many other young women of color into the fold of feminist politics on science, technology, knowledge production and use, and eventually to feminist science and technology studies. So, for very personal and political reasons, I have continued to ask myself how population control is implicated in lifestyle sex selection.

As noted in the introduction, Ikemoto explained how "the population control narrative . . . prepared the ground for claims of entitlement in the family formation and market narratives" that permeate the transnational commercial markets in surrogacy and egg donation (2009, 307). I, too, contend that the preexistence of a population control narrative dovetailed with son preference to condemn sex selection via abortion as "bad." This combined with local anti-abortion politics in the US and UK, and "prepared the ground" for an alternative set of technoscientific practices that could constitute and be defined as "good" by contrast. Yet, it is also within a shifting population control framework that sex selective ART became a set of embodied practices that transform devalued reproducers to reproducers of value in a globalized reproductive economy. Reproducers of value have, of course, already demonstrated rationality and reasonableness by choosing to sex select over endlessly reproducing in the hopes that they will get a child of the desired sex. In this way, they have earned the rights to biocitizenship, which entitles them to the status of an agent free to compose their family as they desire so long as they have requisite wealth. Lifestyle practices, then, constituted not only in opposition to but via abortion, China, India, family limitation, and sex bias.

A feminist research agenda for the future must rethink population control in the context of a new set of powerful ideologies and structures that seek to optimize humans—as separate abstracted entities—in relation to cultural and geographic spaces. Enforced at the individual level of optimizing life itself, biopopulationist interventions can transform formerly targeted objects of population control into consumers within transnational reproductive markets. Yet, the quest to manage individual risks and fulfill individual desires in the realm of reproduction remains tightly interconnected to populationist assumptions—not just about ideal sizes of human units (from family to national populations), but also about ideal forms. Maintaining a feminist critique of population control requires new concepts and a keen understanding of the co-implication of local and global biopolitics.

A meaningful reconceptualization of population control could reenergize an international women's health movement that has at times robustly and at other times haltingly provided an autonomous venue for critical health activism outside the UN. From a first meeting in Rome in 1977 to a twelfth in 2015 in the Dominican Republic, a series of non-affiliated, supranational meetings on women and health built global resistance to targeted and abusive fertility reduction efforts associated with population control. We are in sore need of reviving transnational critical health movements such as these because professional, national, and international mechanisms of governance and accountability to ethics, human rights, and social justice have become increasingly vacuous. Demanding outright bans of sex selection, surrogacy, and a host of other reproductive practices implicated in the production and maintenance of social inequality does not provide a satisfactory solution. Bans remain at best ineffective and at worst part of the "master's tools" either through circumventions that fuel globalized markets or local usurpation by ascendant anti-abortion, right-wing political agendas. However, this does not mean that the best protection for socially marginalized groups lies in succumbing to a libertarian framework of privacy that not only fails to fully protect safe and legal access to abortion but also forces us to abandon other relevant health safety and justice issues, such as those involving sex selection, sterilization, and long-acting contraceptives. We cannot expect effective governance of reproductive technological practices when responsibility for ethical practice shifts to the same institutions that stand to gain commercially from them; this represents a glaring conflict of interest. Transnational critical health movements, informed by the embodied local struggles of people of color, feminists, and queer health activists, can renew pressure on government agencies, professional associations, and international organizations to question the cis- and heteronormative basis for sex selection, *balanced family* as an ideal, and *family balancing* as a rational practice necessarily devoid of bias. Sex selection by whatever means—even when the practices aim to make babies rather than prevent them—and wherever they take place (West or non-West) occurs inside culture and power, and thus is implicated in various kinds of social stratification. To resist these practices as well as the stratification of sex selection itself, we will need to build alternative critical health frameworks that avoid the trap of reproductive binaries as they adapt to shifting transnational terrains.

# Notes

## Introduction

1   Instead of using the individual as a unit of analysis, Adele Clarke focuses
    on social worlds. Emerging from symbolic interactionism, social worlds are
    "meaning-making social groups—collectivities of various sorts" that "gen-
    erate shared perspectives that then form the basis for collective action"
    (Clarke 2005, 45 and 109).
2   I thank Sue Carter for this observation.
3   Feminist theorists in the 1980s and 1990s commonly referred to NRTs,
    or "new reproductive technologies," to mean technologies emerging in the
    late 1970s such as prenatal diagnostic screening techniques and IVF. Using
    "new" as a referent has become increasingly impractical, however, given
    a proliferation of even newer technologies and the construction of bound-
    aries that divide those previously lumped together as "new," such as that
    between prenatal and pre-pregnancy diagnostics, distinguished on the
    basis of whether or not they can avoid tentative pregnancies and abortion
    (Rothman 1993).
4   The Population and Development Program at Hampshire College has taken
    the lead in this effort, bringing together scholars and activists in May 2016
    for an international meeting of thirty-three participants entitled "Old
    Maps, New Terrains: Rethinking Population in an Era of Climate Change."
    At this meeting and through a subsequent collaborative scholarly effort,
    I have joined other feminist scholar/activists working to elaborate a tripar-
    tite conceptual model (demo-, geo- and bio-populationism) to understand
    contemporary interrelated processes of population control (see forthcom-
    ing themed issue of the journal *Gender, Place & Culture*).
5   GIVF did not seek FDA participation and at first challenged it.

## Chapter 1. From Selecting Sexed Sperm and Embryos to Anticipating Lifestyle Sex Selection

1   The term *artificial insemination* (AI) remains current in animal reproductive
    sectors, though it seems to have fallen out of favor in human reproduction.

2   Scientists replaced the cylindrical needle at the flow opening with a beveled needle, directing the stream of sperm cells to flow in a thin ribbon and allowing sperm to orient correctly in the stream. Then, they added a second fluorescence detector at 0° position relative to the laser beam to the standard 90° fluorescence detector. The addition of a second fluorescence detector to the system provided a way to ensure that only properly oriented sperm (as detected by the 90° detector reading the fluorescence intensity of the cell's edge) would be read for fluorescence intensity by the 0° detector (reading the intensity of the cell's face) (Pinkel et al. 1982).

3   Seidel and Garner document the first "heroic experiment" conducted to determine whether the Beltsville Sperm Sexing Technology would work effectively in the cattle industry. Traveling over 1,790 miles by both plane and car, bovine sperm was first collected in Lancaster, PA, during the early morning, driven to the USDA in Beltsville, MD, where it was sorted in five hours and then frozen en route by flight to Denver, CO, with the final destination being Fort Collins, CO. Around midnight the sorted samples were used to inseminate twenty-nine cows (Seidel and Garner 2008, 890).

4   A rushed, same-day purity test was at one point in the clinical trial offered to subjects for an additional fee, but was discontinued due to the logistical difficulties of providing rapid results (IF 9/9/10, IF 12/8/10–12/22/10, Weiss 2007).

5   That is, the process might involve the destruction of healthy embryos.

6   Knowledge of the human chromosomal sex determination system was first articulated in 1905. Both MicroSort and PGD hinge upon the basic knowledge that human sperm, like eggs, are gametes, or reproductive cells, that normally contain twenty-three chromosomes—half the number of a full set of chromosomes. Chromosomes are carriers of genetic material. When sperm combine with egg cells through fertilization, their twenty-three chromosomes are paired with the same number from the egg to make a full set of forty-six pairs. One particular pair, known as the sex chromosomes, is one biological indicator of the sex (female or male) of the developing embryo. Individually identified as either X or Y, sex chromosomes are defined as female, when paired as XX, and as male when paired as XY. Scientists have known since the early twentieth century that because human egg cells always contribute a sex chromosome identified as X and sperm bring either an X- or a Y-bearing chromosome to the pair, the sex chromosome of the sperm decides human sex differentiation.

7   Owned by Gametrics LTD, the Ericsson method can only be used by fertility clinics that pay a licensing fee to Gametrics (their website lists eleven centers in the US, two in Pakistan, and one each in Nigeria, Panama, Colombia, and Egypt), but unlicensed clinics can and do use their own versions of the method (www.childselect.com, accessed on February 23, 2011).

8   As with *high culture*, I use *high* as a referent of taken-for-granted status indicating a more cultivated, advanced, complex, or developed form of

science whose truth and knowledge claims are generally less closely scrutinized.

## Chapter 3. Extending into a Global Market

1  Turkey prohibits travel for reproductive services that involve donor gametes or surrogacy, and New South Wales in Australia has extended extra-territorial application of its ban on commercial surrogacy (Van Hoof and Pennings 2012, 189–190). Scholars of cross-border reproductive care have dubbed these restrictions "unenforceable and largely symbolic" (Inhorn and Patrizio 2012a, 160).

2  Saudi Arabia (Spar 2006); Australia to Thailand to the United States (IF 1/26/11, US clinic B director); Nigeria to South Africa (IF 10/12/10, CEO, Nigerian fertility clinic); Cyprus site of MicroSort laboratory and clinical provision (http://www.microsort.com/?page_id=311); and United Kingdom to Cyprus (Foggo and Newell 2006); Mexico (site of MicroSort laboratory and clinical provision) (http://www.microsort.com/?page_id=311); and satellite location of US clinics offering sex selection (IF 1/24/11, US clinic A director and embryologist); and United States to Mexico (11/19/10 and 11/24/10). The United Arab Emirates is significant generally in cross-border ART (Inhorn and Shrivastav 2010), and MicroSort had an active online recruitment advertisement for a lab technician in Dubai at www.jobsin theuae.com/.

3  Mutlu identifies Northern Cyprus as Turkey's "ethical grey zone." I expand on this idea to refer to jurisdictions where no law or no ethical consensus practically "governs" sex selection as allowable or "not illegal."

4  A recent clinical study demonstrates that day-five biopsies are less harmful to the embryo, increasing chances that it will implant successfully. Unlike on day three, when an embryo only has six to eight cells, day-five embryos have around two hundred cells, and a cell can be extracted from the part of the embryo that will form the placenta, leaving the inner cell mass of the developing fetus intact (Scott et al. 2013).

5  An exception to this is the 2005 statement of the International Federation of Gynecology and Obstetrics (FIGO), which addresses clinics by way of their professional associations. For example, FIGO urges its professional member societies (e.g., ACOG) to "ensure that their members and their staff are accountable for ensuring that their techniques for sex selection are employed only for medical indications" and to "work with their governments to assure that sex selection is strictly regulated" (FIGO 2005). ACOG's 2007 statement on sex selection responded only to the former directive, because, like the ASRM, ACOG supports a system of voluntary "best practices" over government intrusion in clinical practice involving reproductive technologies (Schuppner 2010, 449).

## Chapter 4. Contesting the Known

1 "X-sorts" refer to samples of semen that have undergone the Micro-Sort sperm-sorting process to enrich the number of sperm bearing the X-chromosome so as to increase the chances of having a girl child.

# References

## Interview Files

IF 7/26/10. Interview with nurse at clinic B (US).

IF 8/24/10. Interview with director of clinic A (US).

IF 9/9/10. Interview with director of clinic B (US).

IF 9/14/10. Interview with retired scientist at USDA (US).

IF 10/12/10. Interview with Nigerian clinic director (US).

IF 10/18/10–10/19/10. Interview with campaign representative A (US).

IF 10/19/10. Interview with campaign representative B (US).

IF 10/20/10. Interview with self-help book author A.

IF 10/22/10. Interview with lab technician/administrator in Mexico (US).

IF 11/19/10 and 11/24/10. Interview with clinic director in Mexico (US).

IF 12/8/10–12/22/10. Interview series with scientific director of MicroSort clinical trial (US).

IF 1/24/11. Follow-up interview with director of clinic A (US).

IF 1/24/11. Interview with embryologist at clinic A (US).

IF 1/24/11. Interview with nurse at clinic A (US).

IF 1/26/11. Follow-up interview with director of clinic B (US).

IF 5/28/15. Follow-up interview with MicroSort lab technician/administrator (Mexico).

IF 5/28/15. Interview with traveling embryologist from clinic A (Mexico).

IF 5/29/15. Follow-up interview with traveling director, clinic A (Mexico).

IF 5/29/15. Interview with local director, clinic A (Mexico).

IF 5/29/15. Interview with cryobank director who formerly worked as embryologist in Mexico and North Cyprus (Mexico).

IF 6/3/15. Interview with Norbert Gleicher, the Center for Human Reproduction (New York).

IF 6/22/15. Interview with MicroSort director of international development (US).

IF 7/24/15. Follow-up phone interview with campaign representative A (US).
IF 7/30/15. Interview with campaign representative C (US).

## Fieldnotes

FN 9/10/10. USDA site visit.
FN 10/25/10. ASRM meeting, participant observation (Denver, CO).
FN 1/24/2011. Clinic site visit.
FN 5/27/15. Clinic site visit.

## Secondary Sources

Abrevaya, Joseph. 2009. "Are There Missing Girls in the United States? Evidence for Prenatal Gender Selection." *American Economic Journal: Applied Economics* 1 (2): 1–34.

Abu-Lughod, Lila. [2001] 2013. "*Orientalism* and Middle East Feminist Studies." In *Feminist Theory Reader: Local and Global Perspectives*, 3rd ed., edited by Carole R. McCann and Seung-kyung Kim, 218–226. New York: Routledge.

ACRJ. 2005. "A New Vision for Advancing Our Movement for Reproductive Health, Reproductive Rights and Reproductive Justice." Oakland, CA: Asian Communities for Reproductive Justice (now Forward Together). www.forwardtogether.org/assets/docs/ACRJ-A-New-Vision.pdf.

Adams, Vincanne, Michelle Murphy, and Adele E. Clarke. 2009. "Anticipation: Technoscience, Life, Affect, Temporality." *Subjectivity* 28: 246–265.

Adamson, David. 2005. "Regulation of Assisted Reproductive Technologies in the United States." *Family Law Quarterly* 39 (3): 727–744.

Agigian, Amy. 2007. "Stratified Reproduction." In *The Blackwell Encyclopedia of Sociology*, edited by George Ritzer, 4827–4829. Oxford, UK: Blackwell.

Ahmed, Sara. 2010. "Happy Objects." In *The Affect Theory Reader*, edited by Melissa Gregg and Gregory J. Seigworth, 29–51. Durham, NC: Duke University Press.

———. 2013. "Multiculturalism and the Promise of Happiness." In *Feminist Theory Reader: Local and Global Perspectives*, 3rd ed., edited by Carole R. McCann and Seung-kyung Kim, 517–532. New York: Routledge.

Almond, Douglas, and Lena Edlund. 2008. "Son-Biased Sex Ratios in the 2000 United States Census." *Proceedings of the National Academy of Sciences* 105 (15): 5681–5682. doi:10.1073/pnas.0800703105.

Angus, Ian, and Simon Butler. 2011. *Too Many People? Population, Immigration, and the Environmental Crisis*. Chicago: Haymarket.

Annas, George J. 2011. "Assisted Reproduction: Canada's Supreme Court and the 'Global Baby.'" *New England Journal of Medicine* 365 (5): 459–463.

Asbery, Katherine. 2008. *Altered Dreams . . . Living with Gender Disappointment*. Bloomington, IN: AuthorHouse.

Asch, Adrienne. 1999. "Prenatal Diagnosis and Selective Abortion: A Challenge to Practice and Policy." *American Journal of Public Health* 89 (11): 1649–1657.

Baruch, Susannah. 2008. "Preimplantation Genetic Diagnosis and Parental Preferences: Beyond Deadly Disease." *Houston Journal of Health Law and Policy* 8(2): 245–270.

Baruch, Susannah, David Kaufman, and Kathy L. Hudson. 2008. "Genetic Testing of Embryos: Practices and Perspectives of US In Vitro Fertilization Clinics." *Fertility and Sterility* 89 (5): 1053–1058.

Bazelon, E. "Purvi Patel Could Be Just the Beginning." *New York Times Magazine*, April 1, 2015. www.nytimes.com/2015/04/01/magazine/purvi-patel-could-be-just-the-beginning.html.

Belkin, Lisa. 1999. "Getting the Girl." *New York Times Magazine*, July 25.

Bhatia, Rajani, Rupsa Mallik, and Shamita Das Dasgupta, with contributions from Soniya Munshi and Marcy Darnovsky. 2003. "Sex Selection: New Technologies, New Forms of Discrimination." In *Background Materials on Sex Selection* [distributed at "Within and Beyond Human Nature Conference," Berlin, Germany, October 2003], compiled by Rajani Bhatia, Rupsa Mallik, Marcy Darnovsky, and Shamita Das Dasgupta. http://geneticsandsociety.org/downloads/200308_gupte.pdf.

Birenbaum-Carmeli, Daphna, and Marcia C. Inhorn. 2009. *Assisting Reproduction, Testing Genes: Global Encounters with the New Biotechnologies*. New York: Berghahn.

Bowker, Geoffrey, and Susan Leigh Star. 1999. *Sorting Things Out: Classification and Its Consequences*. Cambridge, MA: MIT Press.

Briggs, Laura. 2010. "Reproductive Technology: Of Labor and Markets." *Feminist Studies* 36 (2): 359–374.

Butler, Judith. 2009. *Frames of War: When Is Life Grievable?* London: Verso.

Callahan, Joan C., ed. 1995. *Reproduction, Ethics, and the Law: Feminist Perspectives*. Bloomington: Indiana University Press.

CDC (Centers for Disease Control and Prevention, American Society for Reproductive Medicine, Society for Assisted Reproductive Technology). 2016. *2014 Assisted Reproductive Technology Fertility Clinic Success Rates Report*. Atlanta: US Department of Health and Human Services.

Chou, Jennifer, and Shivana Jorawar. 2015. "Silently under Attack: AAPI Women and Sex-Selective Abortion Bans." *Asian American Law Journal* 22: 105–117.

CHR (Center for Human Reproduction). 2011. "IVF Clinics Scrambling." www.centerforhumanreprod.com/fertility/ivf-clinics-scrambling/. Accessed July 20, 2015.

Claassens, O. E., C. J. Oosthuizen, J. Brusnicky, D. R. Franken, and T. F. Kruger. 1995. "Fluorescent In Situ Hybridization Evaluation of Human Y-Bearing Spermatozoa Separated by Albumin Density Gradients." *Fertility and Sterility* 63 (2): 417–418.

Clarke, Adele E. 1998. *Disciplining Reproduction: Modernity, American Life Sciences and the "Problems of Sex."* Berkeley: University of California Press.

———. 2005. *Situational Analysis: Grounded Theory after the Postmodern Turn.* Thousand Oaks, CA: Sage.

Clarke, Adele E., Laura Mamo, Jennifer Ruth Fosket, Jennifer R. Fishman, and Janet K. Shim. 2010. *Biomedicalization: Technoscience, Health, and Illness in the U.S.* Durham, NC: Duke University Press.

Clarke, Adele E., Janet K. Shim, Laura Mamo, Jennifer Ruth Fosket, and Jennifer R. Fishman. 2003. "Biomedicalization: Technoscience Transformations of Health, Illness, and U.S. Biomedicine." *American Sociological Review* 68 (2): 161–194.

Committee on Ethics, American College of Obstetricans and Gynecologists. 2007. "ACOG Committee Opinion No. 360: Sex Selection." *Obstetrics and Gynecology* 109 (2, part 1): 475–478.

Committee on Women, Population, and the Environment. 2002. "Letter to J. Benjamin Younger, Executive Director of the American Society for Reproductive Medicine and List of Signatories." *Political Environments*, no. 9. Amherst, MA: Hampshire College, Population and Development Program.

Connelly, Matthew. 2003. "Population Control Is History: New Perspectives on the International Campaign to Limit Population Growth." *Comparative Studies in Society and History* 45 (1): 122–147.

———. 2008. *Fatal Misconception: The Struggle to Control World Population.* Cambridge, MA: Belknap Press of Harvard University Press.

Contractor, Qudsiya, Sumita Menon, and Ravi Duggal. 2003. *Sex Selection Issues and Concerns: A Compilation of Writings.* Mumbai: Centre for Enquiry into Health and Allied Themes.

Corea, Gena, Renate Duelli Klein, Jalna Hanmer, Helen B. Holmes, Betty Hoskins, Madhu Kishwar, Janice Raymond, Robyn Rowland, and Roberta Steinbacher. 1985. *Man-Made Women: How New Reproductive Technologies Affect Women.* London: Hutchinson.

Cornell University Law School Legal Information Institute. n.d. "Title 35–Patents, Part II, Chapter 18, § 209, U.S. Code." www.law.cornell.edu/uscode/35/usc_sec_35_00000209———000-.html. Accessed July 13, 2015.

Croll, Elisabeth. 2000. *Endangered Daughters: Discrimination and Development in Asia.* London. New York: Routledge.

Curtis, Bruce. 2001. *The Politics of Population: State Formation, Statistics, and the Census of Canada, 1840–1875.* Toronto: University of Toronto Press.

Cussins, Charis. 1998. "Producing Reproduction: Techniques of Normalization and Naturalization in Infertility Clinics." In *Reproducing Reproduction: Kinship, Power, and Technological Innovation,* edited by Sarah Franklin and Helena Ragoné, 66–101. Philadelphia: University of Pennsylvania Press.

Darnovsky, Marcy. 2003. "High-Tech Sex Selection." *GeneWatch*, December 31.

Das, Madhab, C. K. Jayaprakasan, Sameer Angras, and Alex C. Varghese. 2013. "Batch In Vitro Fertilization Program." In *A Practical Guide to Setting Up*

*IVF Lab and Embryo Culture Systems and Running the Unit*, edited by Alex C. Varghese, Peter Sjöblum, and K. Jayaprakasan, 181–194. New Delhi: JP Medical Ltd.

Diaz-Tello, F. 2015. "It Is All Too Easy for Pregnant Women to Be Put on Trial in the United States." *RH Reality Check*, March 30. http://rhrealitycheck .org/article/2015/03/30/easy-pregnant-women-put-trial-united-states/.

Dickens, B. M., G. I. Serour, R. J. Cook, and R.-Z. Qiu. 2005. "Sex Selection: Treating Different Cases Differently." *International Journal of Gynaecology and Obstetrics: The Official Organ of the International Federation of Gynaecology and Obstetrics* 90 (2): 171–177.

Dondorp, W., G. De Wert, G. Pennings, F. Shenfield, P. Devroey, B. Tarlatzis, P. Barri, and K. Dietrich. 2013. "Human Reproduction ESHRE Task Force on Ethics and Law 20: Sex Selection for Non-Medical Reasons." *Human Reproduction* 28 (6): 1448–1454.

Eager, Paige Whaley. 2004. *Global Population Policy: From Population Control to Reproductive Rights*. Aldershot, Hants, England: Ashgate.

Edwards, R. G., and H. K. Beard. 1995. "Sexing Human Spermatozoa to Control Sex Ratios at Birth Is Now a Reality." *Human Reproduction* 10 (4): 977–978.

Egan, James, F. X. Winston, A. Campbell, Audrey Chapman, Alireza A. Shamshirsaz, Padmalatha Gurram, and Peter A. Benn. 2011. "Distortions of Sex Ratios at Birth in the United States: Evidence for Prenatal Gender Selection." *Prenatal Diagnosis* 31 (6): 560–565.

ESHRE PGD Consortium Steering Committee. 2002. "ESHRE Preimplantation Genetic Diagnosis Consortium: Data Collection III (May 2001)." *Human Reproduction* 17 (1): 233–246.

Ethics Committee of the American Society for Reproductive Medicine. 1999. "Sex Selection and Preimplantation Genetic Diagnosis." *Fertility and Sterility* 72 (4): 595–598.

———. 2001. "Preconception Gender Selection for Nonmedical Reasons." *Fertility and Sterility* 75 (5): 861–864.

———. 2004. "Preconception Gender Selection for Non-medical Reasons." *Fertility and Sterility* 82 (Suppl. 1). S232–S235.

———. 2015. "Use of Reproductive Technology for Sex Selection for Nonmedical Reasons." *Fertility and Sterility* 103 (6): 1418–1422.

"Family balancing." Dictionary.com. *Collins English Dictionary: Complete and Unabridged 10th Edition*. HarperCollins. http://dictionary.reference.com /browse/family balancing. Accessed July 4, 2015.

"Family Balancing at the Genetics and IVF Institute (GIVF)." 2014. http://bier censl.com/family-balancing-at-the-genetics-ivf-institute-givf/. Accessed July 22, 2015.

FASDSP (Forum against Sex Determination and Sex Preselection). 2003. "Using Technology, Choosing Sex: The Campaign against Sex Determination and the Question of Choice." In *Sex Selection Issues and Concerns: A Compilation of Writings*, edited by Qudsiya Contractor, Sumita Menon, and Ravi Duggal, 7–14. Mumbai: Centre for Enquiry into Health and Allied Themes.

FIGO (International Federation of Gynecology and Obstetrics). 2005. "Resolution on 'Sex Selection for Non-Medical Purposes.'" www.figo.org/projects /sex_selection.

FINRRAGE-UBINIG (Feminist International Network of Resistance to Reproductive and Genetic Engineering–Policy Research for Development Alternatives). 1991. *Declaration of Comila: Proceedings of FINRRAGE-UBINIG International Conference 1989.* Dhaka: UBINIG.

Fishel, Simon, Anthony Gordon, Colleen Lynch, Ken Dowell, George Ndukwe, Ehab Kelada, Simon Thornton, et al. 2010. "Live Birth after Polar Body Array Comparative Genomic Hybridization Prediction of Embryo Ploidy: The Future of IVF?" *Fertility and Sterility* 93 (3): 1006e7–1006e10.

Flaherty, S. P., J. Michalowska, N. J. Swann, W. P. Dmowski, C. D. Matthews, and R. J. Aitken. 1997. "Albumin Gradients Do not Enrich Y-Bearing Human Spermatozoa." *Human Reproduction* 12 (5): 938–942.

Foggo, D., and C. Newell. 2006. "Doctors Offer Illegal Baby Sexing: Couples Pay £12,000 to Get Child of Choice. *Sunday Times,* November 5.

Forums. 2016. "MicroSort in Mexico and Sending Sorted Sample to US Clinic?" *Ingender.com.* www.ingender.com/forum/Thread.aspx?ID=338694.

Foucault, Michel. 1976. *The History of Sexuality. Volume 1: Introduction.* New York: Random House.

Franklin, Sarah. 1997. *Embodied Progress: A Cultural Account of Assisted Conception.* London: Routledge.

Franklin, Sarah, and Celia Roberts. 2006. *Born and Made: An Ethnography of Preimplantation Genetic Diagnosis.* Princeton, NJ: Princeton University Press.

Fraser, Nancy. 2001. "Recognition without Ethics?" *Theory, Culture & Society* 18 (2–3): 21–42.

Fugger, E. F., S. H. Black, K. Keyvanfar, and J. D. Schulman. 1998. "Birth of Normal Daughters after MicroSort Sperm Separation and Intrauterine Insemination, In-Vitro Fertilization, or Intracytoplasmic Sperm Injection." *Human Reproduction* 13 (9): 2367–2370.

Gammelthoft, Tine, and Ayo Wahlberg. 2014. "Selective Reproductive Technologies." *Annual Review of Anthropology* 43 (1): 201–216.

Gandy I. 2015. "Purvi Patel Sentenced to 41 Years for Feticide and Neglect of a Dependent." *RH Reality Check*, March 30. http://rhrealitycheck.org /article/2015/03/30/purvi-patel-sentenced-41-years-feticide-neglect -dependent/. Accessed May 20, 2015.

Gargan, Edward A. 1991. "Ultrasound Skews India's Birth Ratio." *New York Times*, December 13.

Gender Baby. n.d. "Traveling Patients: USA Gender Selection." www.gender -baby.com/traveling-patients/. Accessed June 5, 2017.

"Gender Desire and Disappointment Defined." 2015. www.genderdreaming. com/gender-disappointment/gd-defined/. Accessed July 21, 2015.

"Gender Disappointment." 2007. "Welcome! Please Read Before Posting in This Forum." Online forum message. *Gender Disappointment*. October 26, 2007. www.ingender.com/forum/Thread.aspx?ID=16155. Accessed July 22, 2015.

"Gender Selection for Asians." 2012. Fertility and Gynocology Center, Monterey Bay IVF. www.montereybayivf.com/infertility-services/fertility-services/family-balancing-gender-selection/asian-family/. Accessed July 22, 2015.

Generations Ahead, National Asian Pacific American Women's Forum, and Asian Communities for Reproductive Justice. 2009. *Taking a Stand: Tools for Action on Sex Selection*. www.generations-ahead.org/projects/sex-selection. Accessed March 15, 2016.

Genetics & IVF Institute. 2006. "MicroSort®." http://microsort.net/MicroSort Information.htm. Accessed July 8, 2011.

————. 2013. "Our Founder." www.givf.com/aboutgivf/ourfounder.shtml. Accessed July 13, 2015.

Ghai, Anita. 2002. "Disabled Women: An Excluded Agenda of Indian Feminism." *Hypatia* 17 (3): 49–66.

Gibbon, S., and Novas, C., eds. 2008. *Biosocialities, Genetics and the Social Sciences: Making Biologies and Identities*. New York: Routledge.

Gilbert, D., Walley, T., & New, B. 2000. "Lifestyle Medicines." *British Medical Journal* 321, 1341–1344.

Ginsburg, Faye D., and Rayna Rapp. 1995. *Conceiving the New World Order: The Global Politics of Reproduction*. Berkeley: University of California Press.

Givan, Alice Longobardi. 2001. *Flow Cytometry: First Principles*. New York: Wiley-Liss.

Gleicher, Norbert, and David H. Barad. 2007. "The Choice of Gender: Is Elective Gender Selection, Indeed, Sexist?" *Human Reproduction* 22 (11): 3038–3041.

Gosálvez, J., M. A. Ramirez, C. López-Fernández, F. Crespo, K. M. Evans, M. E. Kjelland, and J. F. Moreno. 2011. "Sex-Sorted Bovine Spermatozoa and DNA Damage: I. Static Features." *Theriogenology* 75 (2): 197–205.

Government of Australia. 2004. *Ethical Guidelines on the Use of Assisted Reproductive Technology [ART] in Clinical Practice and Research*. Paragraph 11.1. www.nhmrc.gov.au/publications/synopses/_files/e78.pdf.

Government of Canada. 2004. *Assisted Human Reproduction Act*, S.C. ch. 2, s. 5(e). http://laws.justice.gc.ca/en/showdoc/cs/A-13.4/bo-ga:s_5/20090616/en#anchorbo-ga:s_5.

Government of India. 1994. *The Pre-Natal Diagnostic Techniques Regulation and Prevention of Misuse Act*. www.india.gov.in/allimpfrms/allacts/2605.pdf.

Government of the People's Republic of China. 1994. *Law on Maternal and Infant Health Care*. www.npc.gov.cn/englishnpc/Law/2007-12/12/content_1383796.htm.

Greenhalgh, Susan. 2003. "Science, Modernity, and the Making of China's One-Child Policy." *Population and Development Review* 29 (2): 163–196.

————. 2010. *Cultivating Global Citizens: Population in the Rise of China*. Cambridge, MA: Harvard University Press.

———. 2013. "Patriarchal Demographics? China's Sex Ratio Reconsidered." *Population and Development Review* 38 (1): 130–149.

Greenhalgh, Susan, and Jiali Li. 1995. "Engendering Reproductive Policy and Practice in Peasant China: For a Feminist Demography of Reproduction." *Signs: Journal of Women in Culture and Society* 20 (3): 601–641.

Greenhalgh, Susan, and Edwin A. Winckler. 2005. *Governing China's Population: From Leninist to Neoliberal Biopolitics.* Stanford, CA: Stanford University Press.

Grewal, Inderpal. 2005. *Transnational America: Feminisms, Diasporas, Neoliberalisms.* Durham, NC: Duke University Press.

Gupte, Manisha. 2003. "A Walk Down Memory Lane: An Insider's Reflection on the Campaign against Sex-Selective Abortions." In *Background Materials on Sex Selection* [distributed at "Within and Beyond Human Nature Conference," Berlin, Germany, October 2003], compiled by Rajani Bhatia, Rupsa Mallik, Marcy Darnovsky, and Shamita Das Dasgupta. http://geneticsand society.org/downloads/200308_gupte.pdf.

Guttmacher Institute. 2016. "Abortion Bans in Cases of Sex or Race Selection or Genetic Anomaly." *Guttmacher Institute.* June 1. www.guttmacher.org/state -policy/explore/abortion-bans-cases-sex-or-race-selection-or-genetic -anomaly. Accessed June 3, 2016.

Hacking, Ian. 1986. "Making Up People." In *Reconstructing Individualism: Autonomy, Individuality, and the Self in Western Thought,* edited by Thomas C. Heller and Christine Brooke-Rose, 222–236. Stanford, CA: Stanford University Press.

Halfmann, Drew. 2011. "Recognizing Medicalization and Demedicalization: Discourses, Practices, and Identities." *Health* 16 (2): 186–207.

Hall, Stuart. 2006. "The West and the Rest: Discourse and Power. In *The Indigenous Experience: Global Perspectives,* edited by Roger C. A. Maaka and Chris Andersen, 165–173. Toronto Canadian Scholars' Press.

Harding, Sandra. 2006. *Science and Social Inequality: Feminist and Postcolonial Issues.* Urbana: University of Illinois Press.

Hartmann, Betsy. 1995. *Reproductive Rights and Wrongs: The Global Politics of Population Control.* Boston: South End Press.

Hecht, Alexander N. 2001. "The Wild Wild West: Inadequate Regulation of Assisted Reproductive Technology." *Houston Journal of Health Law and Policy* 1 (1): 227–261.

Hendrixson, Anne. n.d. "FP2020's '120 by 20' and Implant Access Program: Evidences of Population Control in the Troubled Present." Unpublished manuscript.

HFEA (Human Fertilisation and Embryology Authority). n.d. *HFEA: Code of Practice.* www.hfea.gov.uk/docs/1st_Edition_Code_of_Practice.pdf.

———. 1995. *HFEA: Code of Practice* [revised]. www.hfea.gov.uk/docs/3rd _Edition_Code_of_Practice.pdf.

Holmes, Helen B., and Laura Martha Purdy, eds. 1992. *Feminist Perspectives in Medical Ethics.* Bloomington: Indiana University Press.

Hvistendahl, Mara. 2011. *Unnatural Selection: Choosing Boys over Girls, and the Consequences of a World Full of Men.* New York: PublicAffairs.

Ikemoto, Lisa C. 2009. "Reproductive Tourism: Equality Concerns in the Global Market for Fertility Services." *Law and Inequality: A Journal of Theory and Practice* 27 (2): 277–309.

Ikenberry, G. John. 2008. "The Rise of China and the Future of the West: Can the Liberal System Survive?" *Foreign Affairs*, January/February. www.foreign affairs.com/articles/asia/2008-01-01/rise-china-and-future-west. Accessed December 12, 2016.

Ingender. 2015. "Gender Selection Glossary." http://www.ingender.com/Gender -info/Glossary.aspx. Accessed on July 6, 2015.

Inhorn, Marcia C. 1994. *Quest for Conception: Gender, Infertility, and Egyptian Medical Traditions.* Philadelphia: University of Pennsylvania Press.

———. 2011a. "Globalization and Gametes: Reproductive 'Tourism,' Islamic Bioethics, and Middle Eastern Modernity." *Anthropology & Medicine* 18 (1): 87–103.

———. 2011b. "Diasporic Dreaming: Return Reproductive Tourism to the Middle East." *Reproductive Biomedicine Online* 23: 582–591.

———. 2012. *The New Arab Man: Emergent Masculinities, Technologies, and Islam in the Middle East.* Princeton, NJ: Princeton University Press.

Inhorn, Marcia C., and Aditya Bharadwaj. 2007. "Reproductively Disabled Lives: Infertility, Stigma, and Suffering in Egypt and India." In *Disability in Local and Global Worlds*, edited by Benedicte Ingstad and Susan Reynolds Whyte, 78–106. Berkeley: University of California Press.

Inhorn, Marcia C., and Daphna Birenbaum-Carmeli. 2008. "Assisted Reproductive Technologies and Culture Change." *Annual Review of Anthropology* 37: 177–196.

Inhorn, Marcia C., and Pasquale Patrizio. 2012a. "The Global Landscape of Cross-Border Reproductive Care: Twenty Findings for the New Millennium." *Current Opinion in Obstetrics Gynecology* 24: 158–163.

———. 2012b. "Procreative Tourism: Debating the Meaning of Cross-Border Reproductive Care in the 21st Century." *Expert Review of Obstetrics and Gynecology* 7(6): 509–511.

Inhorn, Marcia C., and P. Shrivastav. 2010. "Globalization and Reproductive Tourism in the United Arab Emirates." *Asia Pacific Journal of Public Health* 22 (3 Suppl.): 68S–74S.

Institute for Human Reproduction. n.d. "Family Balancing." www.infertilityihr .com/family_balancing.html. Accessed June 10, 2015.

Jesudason, Sujatha. n.d. "Attitudes towards and Prevalence of Son Preference and Sex Selection in South Asian American Communities in the United States." www.generations-ahead.org/files-for-download/articles/Genera tionsAhead_SonPreferenceAndSexSelection_(1).pdf. Accessed July 26, 2016.

Jesudason, Sujatha, and Susannah Baruch. n.d. "Race and Sex in Abortion Debates: The Legislation and the Billboards." Generations Ahead. www

.generations-ahead.org/files-for-download/success-stories/RaceAndSex
Selection.pdf. Accessed July 26, 2016.

Johnson, L. A., J. P. Flook, and H. W. Hawk. 1989. "Sex Preselection in Rabbits:
Live Births from X and Y Sperm Separated by DNA and Cell Sorting." *Biology
of Reproduction* 41: 199–203.

Johnson, L. A., J. P. Flook, and M. V. Look. 1987. "Flow Cytometry of X and Y
Chromosome-Bearing Sperm for DNA Using an Improved Preparation
Method and Staining with Hoechst 33342." *Gamete Research* 17: 203–212.

Johnson, L. A., and D. Pinkel. 1986. "Modification of a Laser-Based Flow Cytometer for High Resolution DNA Analysis of Mammalian Spermatazoa."
*Cytometry* 7: 268–273.

Johnson, L. A., and Glenn R. Welch. 1997. "Sex Preselection in Mammals by
DNA: A Method for Flow Separation of X and Y Spermatozoa in Humans."
In *Manual on Assisted Reproduction*, edited by T. Rabe, K. Diedrich, and
B. Runnebaum, 337–349. Berlin: Springer.

Johnson, L. A., Glenn R. Welch, Keyvan Keyvanfar, Andrew Dorfman, Edward
F. Fugger, and Joseph D. Schulman. 1993. "Gender Preselection in Humans?
Flow Cytometric Separation of X and Y Spermatozoa for the Prevention of
X-Linked Diseases." *Human Reproduction* 8 (10): 1733–1739.

Joyce, Christopher. 1999. "Special Delivery." *USA Weekend*, May 14.

Kalantry, Sital. 2014. "Replacing Myths with Facts: Sex-Selective Abortion
Laws in the United States." Cornell Legal Studies Research Paper no. 14–34,
June 5. http://ssrn.com/abstract=2476432.

———. 2015. "Sex-Selective Abortion Bans: Anti-immigration or Anti-
abortion?" *Georgetown Journal of International Affairs* 16 (1): 140–158.

Kalb, Claudia. 2004. "Brave New Babies." *Newsweek*, January 26.

Kaplan, S. 2015. "Indiana Woman Jailed for 'Feticide.' It's Never Happened
Before." *Washington Post*, April 1. www.washingtonpost.com/news/morning
-mix/wp/2015/04/01/indiana-woman-jailed-for-feticide-its-never-hap
pened-before. Accessed May 20, 2015.

Karabinus, David S., Donald P. Marazzo, Harvey J. Stern, Daniel A. Potter,
Chrispo I. Opanga, Marisa L. Cole, Lawrence A. Johnson, and Joseph D.
Schulman. 2014. "The Effectiveness of Flow Cytometric Sporting of Human
Sperm (MicroSort®) for Influencing a Child's Sex." *Reproductive Biology and
Endocrinology* 12 (106): 1–12. www.rbej.com/content/12/1/106: 1–12.

Karst, Kurt R. 2011. "District Court Says 'Shall' Means 'Must' in Challenge to
PTO Denial of Interim Patent Term Extension." www.fdalawblog.net/fda
_law_blog_hyman_phelps/2011/07/district-court-says-shall-means-must
-in-challenge-to-pto-denial-of-interim-patent-term-extension.html.
Accessed July 13, 2015.

Kast, Catherine. 2016. "Chrissy Teigen Shares why She Chose to Have a
Daughter: John Deserves That Bond." *People Magazine*. http://celebrity
babies.people.com/2016/02/24/chrissy-teigen-john-legend-picked-girl
-embryo/. Accessed March 26, 2016.

Kaye, Byron, and Khettiya Jittapong. 2014. "In Thailand Baby Gender Selection Loophole Draws China, HK Women to IVF Clinics." *Reuters*, July 15. www.reuters.com/article/us-thailand-ivf-gender-selection-idUSKBN0FK2H0 20140715.

Klass, Perri. 2001. "Gender Bias." *Vogue*, March, 518–521.

Knecht, Michi, Maren Klotz, and Stefan Beck, eds. 2012. *Reproductive Technologies as Global Form: Ethnographies of Knowledge, Practices, and Transnational Encounters*. Frankfurt: Campus Verlag.

Kolata, Gina. 1998. "Researchers Report Success on Method to Pick Baby's Sex." *New York Times*, September 9. www.nytimes.com/1998/09/09/us/research ers-report-success-in-method-to-pick-baby-s-sex.html.

———. 2001. "Fertility Ethics Authority Approves Sex Selection." *New York Times*, September 28. www.nytimes.com/2001/09/28/us/fertility-ethics -authority-approves-sex-selection.html.

———. 2002. "Fertility Society Opposes Choosing Embryos Just for Sex Selection." *New York Times*, February 16. www.nytimes.com/2002/02/16/us/fer tility-society-opposes-choosing-embryos-just-for-sex-selection.html.

Lambrecht, Petra, and Heide Mertens. 1989. *Small Family Happy Family: Internationale Bevölkerungspolitik und Familienplanung in Indien*. Münster: Verlag Westfälisches Dampfboot.

Lemonick, Michael D. 1999. "Designer Babies." *Time Magazine*, January 11. www.content.time.com/time/magazine/article/0,971,17696,00.html.

Leung, Rebecca. 2004. "Choose the Sex of Your Baby." *60 Minutes*, April 13. www.cbsnews.com/news/choose-the-sex-of-your-baby-13-04-2004/. Accessed June 15, 2017.

Levinson, G., K. Keyvanfar, J. C. Wu, E. F. Fugger, R. A. Fields, L. Calvo, R. J. Sherins, D. Bick, J. D. Schulman, and S. H. Black. 1995. "DNA-Based X-Enriched Sperm Separation as an Adjunct to Preimplantation Genetic Testing for the Prevention of X-Linked Disease. *Human Reproduction* 10 (4): 979–982.

Levsky, Jeffrey M., and Robert H. Singer. 2003. "Fluorescence in Situ Hybridization: Past, Present and Future." *Journal of Cell Science* 116: 2833–2838.

Lohmann, Larry. 2005. "Malthusianism and the Terror of Scarcity." In *Making Threats: Biofears and Environmental Anxieties*, edited by Betsy Hartmann, Banu Subramaniam, and Charles Zerner. Lanham, MD: Rowman and Littlefield.

Lorde, Audre. [1979] 2015. "The Master's Tools Will Never Dismantle the Master's House." In *This Bridge Called My Back: Writings by Radical Women of Color*, (4th ed.), edited by Cherrie Moraga and Gloria Anzaldúa, 94–103. Albany: SUNY Press.

Luna, Zaikiya, and Kristin Luker. 2013. "Reproductive Justice." *Annual Review of Law and Social Science* 9: 327–352.

Mallik, Rupsa. 2003. *"Negative Choice" Sex Determination and Sex Selective Abortion in India*. Mumbai: Centre for Enquiry into Health and Allied Themes.

Mamo, Laura. 2007. *Queering Reproduction: Achieving Pregnancy in the Age of Technoscience*. Durham, NC: Duke University Press.

———. 2010. "Consumption and Subjectification in U.S. Lesbian Reproductive Practices." In *Biomedicalization: Technoscience, Health, and Illness*, edited by Adele E. Clarke, Laura Mamo, Jennifer Ruth Fosket, Jennifer R. Fishman, and Janet K. Shim, 173–196. Durham, NC: Duke University Press.

Mamo, Laura, and Jennifer R. Fishman. 2013. "Why Justice?: Introduction to the Special Issue on Entanglements of Science, Ethics, and Justice." *Science, Technology, and Human Values* 38 (2): 1–17.

Marazzo, Donald P., David Karabinus, Lawrence A. Johnson, and Joseph D. Schulman. 2015. "MicroSort® Sperm Sorting Causes No Increase in Major Malformation Rate." *Reproduction, Fertility and Development*. http://dx .doi.org/10.1071/RD15011.

Mazumdar, Vina. 1991. "Declining Sex Ratio: A View from the Women's Movement." Paper 13. In *Symposium on the 1991 Census of India: Methodology and Implications of First Results*. New Delhi: Population and Research Centre, Institute of Economic Growth."

Mbembe, Achille. 2003. "Necropolitics." *Public Culture* 15 (1): 11–40.

McCann, Carole. 2009. "Malthusian Men and Demographic Transitions: A Case Study of Hegemonic Masculinity in Mid-Twentieth-Century Population Theory." *Frontiers: A Journal of Women's Studies* 30 (1): 142–171.

McGowan, Michelle L., and Richard R. Sharp. 2013. "Justice in the Context of Family Balancing." *Science, Technology, and Human Values* 38 (2): 271–293.

Medstar LLC. 2010. "MicroSort (Gender Selection)." Mexico City. http://www .whereismy doctor.com/infertility-ivf-specialists/microsort-gender-selection /mexico/mexico- city. Accessed September 20, 2011.

Menon, Nivedita. 1995. "The Impossibility of 'Justice': Female Foeticide and Feminist Discourse on Abortion." *Contributions to Indian Sociology* 29 (1–2): 369–392.

Mies, Maria. 1991. "What Unites, What Divides Women from the North and the South in the Field of Reproductive Technologies." In *Declaration of Comila: Proceedings of FINRRAGE-UBINIG International Conference 1989*, edited by Farida Akhter, Wilma van Berkel, and Natasha Ahmad, 33–43. Dhaka: UBINIG.

Miller, Korin. 2016, February 29. "Chrissy Teigen and John Legend Chose the Sex of Their Baby—Here's How That's Possible," *Self Magazine*. www.self .com/trending/2016/02/chrissy-teigen-and-john-legend-chose-the-sex-of -their-baby-heres-how-thats-possible/. Accessed July 25, 2016.

Mohanty, Chandra Talpade. 2003. *Feminism without Borders: Decolonizing Theory, Practicing Solidarity*. Durham, NC: Duke University Press.

Morales, Tatiana. 2002. "Choosing Your Baby's Gender." *The Early Show*. November 6. www.cbsnews.com/news/choosing-you-babys-gender/. Accessed June 15, 2017.

Murphy, Michelle. 2012. *Seizing the Means of Reproduction: Entanglements of Feminism, Health, and Technoscience.* Durham, NC: Duke University Press.

Mutlu, Burcu. 2015. "The Gendered Ethics of Secrecy and Disclosure in Transnational Sex Selection from Turkey to Northern Cyprus." In *(In)Fertile Citizens: Anthropological and Legal Challenges of Assisted Reproductive Technologies,* edited by Venetia Kantsa, Giulia Zanini, and Lina Papadopoulou, 217–229. Mytilene: (In)FERCIT, University of the Aegean.

Napoli, Lisa. 2006. "I'll Have a Girl, Please." *Marketplace,* September 12.

NAPAWF (National Asian Pacific American Women's Forum). 2005. "Sex Selection: A Fact Sheet." https://napawf.org/wp-content/uploads/2009/working /pdfs/sex_selection_factsheet.pdf. Accessed June 13, 2016.

———. 2015. "Factsheet: NAACP & NAPAWF vs. Tom Horne." https://napawf .org/newsroom/press-releases-statements/naacp-and-napawf-v-arizona/. Accessed March 20, 2016.

———. 2013. "Race and Sex Selective Abortion Bans: Wolves in Sheep's Clothing." Issue brief. https://napawf.org/wp-content/uploads/2009/10/PRENDA IssueBrief_8.5_Final.pdf. Accessed June 13, 2016.

———. 2015. "Webinar: NAACP & NAPAWF v. Tom Horne." Webinar. www .youtube.com/watch?v=IrkI7RmtRE8&feature=youtu.be&can_id=&source =email-thank-for-attending-naacp-napawf-v-tom-horne-webinar-panel& email_referrer=thank-for-attending-naacp-napawf-v-tom-horne-webinar -panel. Accessed June 7, 2016.

Narayan, Uma. 1997. *Dislocating Cultures: Identities, Traditions, and Third World Feminism.* New York: Routledge.

Ogilvie, C. M., Peter R. Braude, and and Paul N. Scriven. 2005. "Preimplantation Genetic Diagnosis: An Overview." *Journal of Histochemistry and Cytochemistry* 53 (3): 255–260.

Ong, Aihwa. 1999. *Flexible Citizenship: The Cultural Logics of Transnationality.* Durham, NC: Duke University Press.

Ong, Aihwa, and Stephen J. Collier. 2005. *Global Assemblages: Technology, Politics, and Ethics as Anthropological Problems.* Malden, MA: Blackwell.

Ouellette, Alicia, Arthur Caplan, Kelly Carroll, James W. Fossett, Dyrleif Bjarnadottir, Darren Shickle, and Glenn McGee. 2005. "Lessons across the Pond: Assisted Reproductive Technology in the United Kingdom and the United States." *American Journal of Law and Medicine* 31 (4): 419–446.

Overall, Christine. 1987. "Book Review." *Canadian Journal of Philosophy* 17 (3): 683–692.

Oviedo Convention. 1997. European Convention on Human Rights and Biomedicine, Article 14. 1997. www.coe.int/t/dg3/healthbioethic/Activities/01 _Oviedo%20Convention/.

Paltrow, L. 2015. "How Indiana Is Making It Possible to Jail Women for Having Abortions." *Political Research Associates.* March 29. www.politicalresearch

.org/2015/03/29/how-indiana-is-making-it-possible-to-jail-women-for
-having-abortions/#sthash.Ra5sWeAf.dpbs. Accessed May 20, 2015.

Paltrow, L. M., and J. Flavin. 2013. "The Policy and Politics of Reproductive
Health: Arrests of and Forced Interventions on Pregnant Women in the
United States, 1973–2005: Implications for Women's Legal Status and
Public Health." *Journal of Health Politics, Policy and Law* 38 (2): 299–343.
doi: 10.1215/03616878–1966324.

Pande, Amrita. 2014. *Wombs in Labor: Transnational Commercial Surrogacy in
India*. New York: Columbia University Press.

Patel, Tulsi. 2007. *Sex-Selective Abortion in India: Gender, Society and New Reproductive Technologies*. New Delhi: Sage.

Penketh R., and A. McLaren. 1987. "Prospects for Prenatal Diagnosis during
Preimplantation Human Development." *Baillière's International Clinical
Obstetrics and Gynaecology* 1: 747–764.

Pennings, Guido. 1996. "Ethics of Sex Selection for Family Balancing." *Human
Reproduction* 11 (11): 2339–2345.

———. 2004. "Legal Harmonization and Reproductive Tourism in Europe."
*Human Reproduction* 19 (12): 2689–2694.

———. 2009. "International Evolution of Legalisation and Guidelines in Medically Assisted Reproduction." *Reproductive BioMedicine Online* 18 (Suppl. 2):
S15–S19. www.rbmonline.com/Article/3783.

Perwez, Shahid, Roger Jeffery, and Patricia Jeffrey. 2012. "Declining Sex Ratio
and Sex-Selection in India: A Demographic Epiphany." *Economic and Political
Weekly* 18: 47 (33): 73–77.

Petchesky, Rosalind P. 1990 [1984]. *Abortion and Woman's Choice: The State, Sexuality, and Reproductive Freedom*. Rev. ed. Boston: Northeastern University Press.

———. 2003. *Global Prescriptions: Gendering Health and Human Rights*. London:
Zed Books.

Pinkel, D., S. Lake, B. L. Gledhill, M. A. Van Dilla D. Stephenson, and G. Watch-
maker. 1982. "High Resolution DNA Content Measurements of Mammalian
Sperm." *Cytometry* 3 (1): 1–9.

Platoni, Kara. 2004. "It's a Boy! We Made Sure of It." *East Bay Express*, November 3.

PRWeb 2015. "Advanced Gender Selection Program Announced at LIV Fertility
Center in Mexico." www.prweb.com/releases/liv-ivf-mexico/gender-selection
/prweb12475235.htm.

Purdy, Laura. 2007. "Is Preconception Sex Selection Necessarily Sexist?" *Reproductive Biomedicine Online* 15 (Suppl. 2): 33–37.

Purewal, Navtek K. 2010. *Son Preference, Gender and Culture in South Asia*. New
York: Berg.

Puri, Sunita, Vincanne Adams, Susan Ivey, and Robert D. Nachtigall. 2011.
"'There Is Such a Thing as Too Many Daughters, but not Too Many Sons': A
Qualitative Study of Son Preference and Fetal Sex Selection among Indian
Immigrants in the United States." *Social Science and Medicine* 72 (7): 1169–1176.

Rabinow, Paul. 1996. *Making PCR: A Story of Biotechnology.* Chicago: University of Chicago Press.

Ragoné, Helena, and Sarah Franklin. 1998. *Reproducing Reproduction: Kinship, Power, and Technological Innovation.* Philadelphia: University of Pennsylvania Press.

Rainsbury Clinic. n.d. "Freedom to Ask." www.gender-baby.com/traveling-patients/. Accessed June 25, 2016.

Rao, Mohan, and Sarah Sexton. 2010. *Markets and Malthus: Gender, Population and Health in Neoliberal Times.* New Delhi: Sage.

Ravindra, R. P. 1993. "The Campaign against Sex Determination Tests." In *The Struggle against Violence*, edited by Chhaya Datar, 51–99. Calcutta: Shree.

Raymond, Janice. 1981. "Introduction, Sex Preselection." In *The Custom-Made Child?: Women-Centered Perspectives*, edited by Helen B. Holmes, Betty B. Hoskins, and Michael Gross, 177–180. New York: Humana Press.

Raymond, Janice. 1993. *Women as Wombs: Reproductive Technologies and the Battle over Women's Freedom.* San Francisco: Harper.

Revesz, Rachael. 2016. "Purvi Patel: Judge Orders Release of Woman Given 20 Years for Rare Crime of Feticide." *Independent*, September 1. www.independent.co.uk/news/world/americas/purvi-patel-feticide-freed-released-prison-indiana-20-year-sentence-a7220251.html.

Riessman, Catherine K. 1983. "Women and Medicalization: A New Perspective." *Social Policy* 14 (1): 3–18.

Roberts, Dorothy. 1997. *Killing the Black Body: Race, Reproduction and the Meaning of Liberty.* New York: Vintage Books.

———. 2009. "Race, Gender, and Genetic Technologies: A New Reproductive Dystopia?" *Signs: Journal of Women in Culture and Society* 34 (4): 783–804.

Robertson, John. 1998. "Liberty, Identity, and Human Cloning." *Texas Law Review* 76 (6): 1390–1391.

———. 2001. "Preconception Gender Selection." *American Journal of Bioethics* 1 (1): 2–9.

———. 2003. "Extending Preimplantation Genetic Diagnosis: Medical and Non-Medical Uses." *Journal of Medical Ethics* 29 (4): 213–216.

Rose, G. A., and A. Wong. 1998. "Experiences in Hong Kong with the Theory and Practice of the Albumin Column Method of Sperm Separation for Sex Selection." *Human Reproduction* 13 (1): 146–149.

Rose, Nikolas. 2006. *Politics of Life Itself: Biomedicine, Power and Subjectivity in the Twenty-First Century.* Princeton, NJ: Princeton University Press.

Rose, Nikolas, and Carlos Novas. 2005. "Biological Citizenship." In *Global Assemblages: Technology, Politics and Ethics as Anthropological Problems*, edited by Aihwa Ong and Stephen J. Collier, 439–463. Malden, MA: Blackwell.

Rosin, Hanna. 2010. "The End of Men." *Atlantic*. July/August.

Rothman, Barbara Katz. 1993. *The Tentative Pregnancy: How Amniocentesis Changes the Experience of Motherhood.* New York: Norton.

Rubin, Gayle. [1975] 1997. "The Traffic in Women: Notes on the 'Political

Economy' of Sex." In *The Second Wave: A Reader in Feminist Theory,* edited by Linda Nicholson, 27–62. New York: Routledge.

Rudruppa, Sharmila. 2015. *Discounted Life: The Price of Global Surrogacy in India.* New York: New York University Press.

Sachs, Susan. 2001. "Clinics' Pitch to Indian Émigrés." *New York Times.* August 15.

Saharso, Sawitri. 2003. "Feminist Ethics, Autonomy and the Politics of Multiculturalism." *Feminist Theory* 4 (2): 199–215.

SAMA–Resource Group for Women and Health. 2005. *Beyond Numbers: Implications of the Two-Child Norm.* New Delhi: SAMA–Resource Group for Women and Health.

Schake, Kori, and Anja Manuel. 2016. "How to Manage a Rising Power—or Two: What America Can Learn from 19th Century Britain." *Atlantic,* May 24. www .theatlantic.com/international/archive/2016/05/china-india-rising-powers /484106/. Accessed December 12, 2016.

Schulman, Joseph D. 1993. "Ethical Issues in Gender Selection by X/Y Sperm Separation." *Human Reproduction* 8 (10): 1541.

———. 2007. *Why Do Bad Investments Happen to Smart People?* XLIBRIS Corp.

———. 2010. *Robert G. Edwards: A Personal Viewpoint.* CreateSpace Independent Publishing Platform.

Schulman, Joseph D., and David S. Karabinus. 2005. "Scientific Aspects of Preconception Gender Selection." *Reproductive Biomedicine Online* 10: 111–115.

Schultz, Susanne. 2010. "Redefining and Medicalizing Population Policies." In *Markets and Malthus: Population, Gender, and Health in Neo-liberal Times,* edited by Mohan Rao and Sarah Sexton, 173–214. New Delhi: Sage.

———. 2015. "Reproducing the Nation: The New German Population Policy and the Concept of Demographization." *Distinktion: Skandinavian Journal of Social Theory* 16 (3): 337–361.

Schuppner, Nicole C. 2010. "Preimplantation Genetic Diagnosis: A Call for Public Sector Implementation of Private Advocacy Regulation." *Michigan State Journal of International Law* 14 (2): 443–455.

Scott, Richard T., Kathleen M. Upham, Eric J. Forman, Kathleen H. Hong, Katherine L. Scott, Deanne Taylor, Xin Tao, and Nathan R. Treff. 2013. "Blastocyst Biopsy with Comprehensive Chromosome Screening and Fresh Embryo Transfer Significantly Increases In Vitro Fertilization Implantation and Delivery Rates: A Randomized Controlled Trial." *Fertility and Sterility* 100 (3): 697–703.

Seavilleklein, Victoria, and Susan Sherwin. 2007. "The Myth of the Gendered Chromosome: Sex Selection and the Social Interest." *Cambridge Quarterly of Healthcare Ethics* 16 (1): 7–19.

Seidel, G. E., Jr., with D. L. Garner. 2008. "History of Commercializing Sexed Semen for Cattle." *Theriogenology* 69: 886–895.

Sen, Amartya. 1990. "More than 100 Million Women Are Missing." *New York Review of Books,* December 20, 61–66.

Sen, Gita, Adrienne Germain, and Lincoln C. Chen, eds. 1994. *Population Policies Reconsidered: Health, Empowerment, and Rights*. Boston: Harvard Center for Population and Development Studies.

Sermon, Karen, Andre Van Steirteghem, and Inge Liebaers. 2004. "Preimplantation Genetic Diagnosis." *Lancet* 363: 1633–1641.

Sexing Technologies LLC. 2012. "History." www.sexingtechnologies.com/articles/history. Accessed March 20, 2015.

Sherins, R. J., L. P. Thorsell, A. Dorfmann, L. Dennison-Lagos, L. P. Calvo, L Krysa, C. B. Coulam, and J. D. Schulman. 1995. "Intracytoplasmic Sperm Injection Facilitates Fertilization Even in the Most Severe Forms of Male Infertility: Pregnancy Outcome Correlates with Maternal Age and Number of Eggs Available." *Fertility and Sterility* 64 (2): 369–375.

Silliman, Jael, and Anannya Bhattacharjee. 2002. *Policing the National Body: Race, Gender, and Criminalization*. Boston: South End Press.

Silliman, Jael, Marlene Gerber Fried, Loretta Ross, and Elena Gutierrez. 2004. *Undivided Rights: Women of Color Organize for Reproductive Justice*. Boston: South End Press.

Simon-Kumar, Rachel. 2010. "Neo-liberal Development and Reproductive Health in India: The Making of the Personal and the Political." In *Markets and Malthus: Population, Gender, and Health in Neo-liberal Times*, edited by Mohan Rao and Sarah Sexton, 127–155. Thousand Oaks, CA: Sage.

Singh, Abhishek, Reuben Ogollah, Faujdar Ram, and Saseendran Pallikadavath. 2012. "Sterilization Regret among Married Women in India: Implications for the Indian National Family Planning Program." *International Perspectives on Sexual and Reproductive Health* 38 (4): 187–195.

Spar, Debora L. 2006. *The Baby Business: How Money, Science and Politics Drive the Commerce of Conception*. Boston: Harvard Business School Press.

Stapleton, Patricia. 2015. "The Inauspicious Regulatory Beginnings of Preimplantation Genetic Diagnosis." In *Biopolitics and Utopia: An Interdisciplinary Reader*, edited by Patricia Stapleton and Andrew Byers, 63–86. New York: Palgrave MacMillan.

Steel, Tanya Wenman. 2003. "Would You (Should You) Choose Your Baby's Sex?" *Child*, December–January.

Steinbock, Bonnie. 2002. "Sex Selection: Not ♂bviously Wr♀ng." *Hastings Center Report* 32 (1): 23–28.

Strathern, Marilyn. 1992. *Reproducing the Future: Essays on Anthropology, Kinship, and the New Reproductive Technologies*. New York: Routledge.

Takeshita, Chikako. 2012. *Global Biopolitics of the IUD*. Cambridge, MA: MIT Press.

Tambe A. 2015. "The Indiana Foeticide Case: Why Purvi Patel's Indianness Matters." *Scroll.in*, April 11. http://scroll.in/article/718081/the-indiana-foeticide-case-why-purvi-patels-indianness-matters.

Theodosiou, Anastasia A., and Martin H. Johnson. 2011. "The Politics of Human Embryo Research and the Motivation to Achieve PGD." *Reproductive BioMedicine Online* 22 (5): 457–471.

Thompson, Charis. 2005. *Making Parents: The Ontological Choreography of Reproductive Technologies*. Cambridge, MA: MIT Press.

Thompson, Jennifer Merrill. 2004. *Chasing the Gender Dream*. Chula Vista, CA: Aventine Press.

Ticktin, Miriam. 2005. "Culture or Inequality in Sex-Selective Abortion? A Response to Sawriti Saharso." *Ethnicities* 5 (2): 266–271.

UBINIG (Policy Research for Development Alternatives). 1993. "The Declaration of People's Perspectives on 'Population' Symposium." Comilla, Bangladesh, December 12–15.

UNFPA (United Nations Population Fund). 1995. "Report of the International Conference on Population and Development." www.un.org/popin/icpd/conference/offeng/poa.html. Accessed June 15, 2017.

———. 2011. "Gender at the Heart of ICPD: The UNFPA Strategic Framework on Gender Mainstreaming and Women's Empowerment." www.unfpa.org/publications/gender-heart-icpd. Accessed June 15, 2017.

UN Women. 1996. "Report of the Fourth World Conference on Women." www.un.org/womenwatch/daw/beijing/official.htm.

———. 2014. *Sex Ratios and Gender Biased Sex Selection: History, Debates and Future Directions*. New Delhi: UN Women.

US Department of Agriculture. 2008. "License Application Instructions for Patents or Pending Patents." www.ars.usda.gov/SP2UserFiles/Place/00000000/LicensingInfo/InstructionsforPatents.3.17.08.pdf. Accessed July 13, 2015.

US Food and Drug Administration. 2010. "Genetics & IVF Institute IRB 12/23/09." *Inspections, Compliance, Enforcement, and Criminal Investigations*. www.fda.gov/ICECI/EnforcementActions/WarningLetters/ucm203906.htm. Accessed July 22, 2015.

———. 2015a. "Genetics & IVF Institute, 11/20/09." *Inspections, Compliance, Enforcement, and Criminal Investigations*. www.fda.gov/ICECI/EnforcementActions/WarningLetters/ucm193908.htm. Accessed July 13, 2015.

———. 2015b. "Potter, Daniel A., M.D." *Inspections, Compliance, Enforcement, and Criminal Investigations*. www.fda.gov/ICECI/EnforcementActions/WarningLetters/ucm197438.htm. Accessed July 13, 2015.

Van Dilla, M. A., B. L. Gledhill, S. Lake, P. N. Dean, J. W. Gray, V. Kachel, B. Barlogie, and W. Göhde. 1977. "Measurement of Mammalian Sperm Deoxyribonucleic Acid by Flow Cytometry: Problems and Approaches." *Journal of Histochemistry and Cytochemistry* 25 (7): 763–773.

Van Hoof, Wannes, and Guido Pennings. 2011. "Extraterritoriality for Cross-Border Reproductive Care: Should States Act against Citizens Travelling Abroad for Illegal Infertility Treatment?" *Reproductive BioMedicine Online* 23 (5): 546–554.

———. 2012. "Extraterritorial Laws for Cross-Border Reproductive Care: The Issue of Legal Diversity." *European Journal of Health Law* 19 (2): 187–200.

Varghese, Philip. 2011. "'Abortion Is not Murder,' Says Letter to Speaker." *After-*

noon *Despatch and Courier Mumbai*, August 10. www.afternoondc.in/city
-news/abortion-is-not-murder-says-letter-to-speaker/article_32044.

Visaria, Leela. 2007. "Deficit of Girls in India: Can It Be Attributed to Female
Selective Abortion?" In *Sex-Selective Abortion in India: Gender, Society and
New Reproductive Technologies*, edited by Tulsi Patel, 61–79. New Delhi: Sage.

Wadman, Meredith. 2001. "So You Want a Girl? A New Technology Lets Parents
Order Up the Sex of Their Child. It's Poised to Become Big Business—and a
Big Ethical Dilemma." *Fortune*, February 19. http://money.cnn.com/maga
zines/fortune/fortune_archive/2001/02/19/296875/.

Waldby, Catherine, and Melinda Cooper. 2010. "From Reproductive Work to
Regenerative Labor: The Female Body and the Stem Cell Industries." *Feminist Theory* 11(1): 3–22.

Warren, Mary Anne. 1985. *Gendercide: The Implications of Sex Selection*. Totowa,
NJ: Rowman and Allanheld.

Weaver-Missick, Tara. 1999. "New Accuracy in Sex Selection." *Agricultural
Research Magazine* 47 (5): 12–13.

Weiss, Robin Elise. 2007. *Guarantee the Sex of Your Baby*. Berkeley: Ulysses Press.

Westhorp, Tanya. 2013. "Couples Go to Asia to Select Baby Gender." *Gold Coast
Bulletin*, April 2. www.news.com.au/lifestyle/parenting/couples-go-to-asia
-to-select-baby-gender/story-fneto8ck-1226610697956.

Whittaker, A. M., 2011. "Reproductive Opportunists in the New Global Sex
Trade: PGD and Non-medical Sex Selection." *Reproductive BioMedicine
Online* 23: 609–617.

———. 2012. "Gender Disappointment and Cross-Border High-Tech Sex Selection: A New Global Sex Trade." In *Technologies of Sexuality, Identity and Sexual Health*, edited by Leonore Manderson, 143–164. New York: Routledge.

WHO. 2011. *Preventing Gender-Biased Sex Selection: An Interagency Statement*.
www.who.int/reproductivehealth/publications/gender_rights/9789241501460
/en.

Wilkinson, Stephen, and Eve Garrard. 2013. *Eugenics and the Ethics of Selective
Reproduction*. Keele, UK: Keele University. www.keele.ac.uk/media/keele
university/ri/risocsci/eugenics2013/Eugenics%20and%20the%20ethics%20
of%20selective%20reproduction%20Low%20Res.pdf.

Wilson, Kalpana. 2012. *Race, Racism and Development: Interrogating History,
Discourse and Practice*. London: Zed Books.

World Economic Forum. 2015. "The Global Gender Gap Report 2015." www
.reports.weforum.org/global-gender-gap-report-2015/.

Xinhua. 2016. "Chinese Couples Flock to Thailand for Cheap IVF, Illicit Gender
Selection." *Global Times*, January 21. www.globaltimes.cn/content/965977
.shtml.

# Index

Ahmed, Sara, 102, 104, 106, 114

All-India Institute of Medical Sciences, 65

Almond, Douglas, 162, 163, 164, 166, 169, 182

*Altered Dreams: Living with Gender Disappointment* (Asbery), 107

American Civil Liberties Union (ACLU), 170

American Medical Association (AMA), 64

American Psychiatric Association, 108

Americans, cultural stereotypes, 109–10, 111. *See also* West/Rest binary

American Society for Reproductive Medicine (ASRM), 92, 167, 197; Ethics Committee approval for sex selection via PGD, 6, 89, 158–59; Ethics Committee statements, 85–89, 93–95, 150, 185

Americans United for Life, 162–63

amniocentesis, 24, 47, 64–65, 69

Andolan–Organizing South Asian Workers, 159

Angus, Ian, 27

animals. *See* agricultural industry

Annas, George, 78

ANSIRH (Advancing New Standards in Reproductive Health), 168–69, 180

anti-abortion activism, 5, 70, 71, 192; campaign activists against, 7, 160, 162–64, 166, 168–70, 173–74, 180–81; India law and, 175; against PGD, 46–48, 65; race and, 7, 17, 32, 166, 173, 181, 191; rhetoric in, 170, 177–79, 198; RJ and, 198–99; sex selection bans proposed, 162–63, 168–70, 175, 203; truth claims and knowledge production, 15–16, 163, 166, 168–70; West/Rest binary and, 188, 191. *See also* abortion; "the campaign" (sex selection activism), history of; sex selective abortion;

sex selective abortion bans; sex selective abortion bans, race and

Apna Ghar, 176

artificial insemination (AI), 41, 55, 57, 205n1. *See also* intrauterine insemination (IUI); in vitro fertilization (IVF)

Asbery, Katherine, 99, 106, 107

Asch, Adrienne, 11

Asian Americans, 32, 160, 198; feticide law and, 174–75; Patel case, 174, 175–78; "Replacing Myths," 168–70, 180, 182, 186, 187–88; sex ratios and, 162, 164, 169, 183; sex selective abortion bans and, 171–72, 174

Asian American stereotypes, 166, 171, 174, 176, 180, 190; sex bias, 155, 163, 169, 183. *See also* Orientalism

Asian Communities for Reproductive Justice (ACRJ), 164, 166, 172

ASRM. *See* American Society for Reproductive Medicine (ASRM)

assisted reproductive technology (ART), defined, 4, 9–10

*Atlantic* magazine, 154

Australia, 117, 119, 122, 123, 207n1

babycenter.com, 107

Baruch, Susannah, 90, 164

Beard, Helen K., 56, 58

Beijing Declaration and Platform of Action, 149

Belkin, Lisa, 103–4, 104–5, 106, 109

Beltsville Sperm Sexing Technology (later MicroSort), 33, 40–45, 50–55, 62, 80, 206n3. *See also* MicroSort

beta-thalassemia, 48–49

BGI (Chinese genomics firm), 131

bio- (prefix), 26–27

biocitizenship, 95, 111–14, 121–22, 197–98, 202; of biopolitical subjects, 31, 110; construction of, 16, 25–26

crossover applications of sex selection, 36, 93–94, 123, 150–51, 155–57
cryopreservation: of embryos, 132, 138–39; of sperm, 36, 61, 127–28, 130
cultural economies, 14, 32, 194
Curtis, Bruce, 26
Cussins, Charis, 60
CWPE (Committee on Women, Population, and the Environment), 158, 159
Cyprus, 119, 124, 126, 141, 207n3
cytometry. *See* flow cytometry

data collection (raw data), 16; Almond and Edlund study, 162; campaign goal to increase published, 161, 164–65, 166, 168, 197; campaign's reservations about, 165–66, 168; context of, 181, 190; limiting factors, 153–57; in MicroSort clinical trials, 5, 80, 82, 94, 142, 154, 164–66; on PGD, 5, 154–57; sex ratios, 164, 165, 168, 169, 181–83; sex selective abortion, 153, 165–66, 168–75. *See also* "the campaign" (sex selection activism), data and; knowledge production and truth claims (data interpretation)
daughters. *See* female selection
Day, Doris, 13
desire. *See* individual desire
devalued reproduction, 171, 177, 202; valued reproduction, 16–17, 20, 202
developing countries, population control in. *See* China; India; population control; West/Rest binary
Diagnostic and Statistical Manual (DSM-IV), 108
disadvantaged groups, RJ activism and, 153, 171–72, 173, 174
*Disciplining Reproduction* (Clarke), 63
discrimination. *See* Orientalism; race; sex bias

disease prevention. *See* genetic disease prevention
dissociation from abortion. *See* sex selective abortion, dissociation from
divisible sex selection process. *See* reproductive travelers, interclinic collaboration
DNA: amplification/reproduction, 48; content in human sperm, 50, 51, 52, 54; FISH and, 35–36; flow cytometry and, 33, 34–35, 43; PGD and, 35–36, 49
doctors. *See* providers
Dorfman, Andrew, 45
dye staining, 34–35, 43, 52, 54. *See also* fluorescence in situ hybridization (FISH)

Eager, Paige Whaley, 25–26
economic recession (2008), 90
Edlund, Lena, 162, 163, 164, 166, 169, 182
Edwards, Robert, 40, 41, 56, 58
Egan, James, 163
egg donation, 31, 117, 119, 202
elective interventions. *See* biomedicalized sex selection
embryo analysis, 4–5; biopsy, 35–36, 41, 131–33, 135, 146–47, 207n4; micro-array CGH, 36, 93, 132, 133, 156–57. *See also* fluorescence in situ hybridization (FISH); preimplantation genetic diagnosis (PGD)
embryo freezing, 132, 138–39
embryo production, ethical concerns, 65–66, 67, 85, 206n5; research and, 78; vs. sperm sexing, 33, 58, 124
embryo production through IVF, 5, 48, 60; increasing female embryos, 37, 56; legality and reproductive travel, 118, 125; staggered cycles, 36, 132, 138. *See also* in vitro fertilization (IVF)

embryo research: ethical debates, 78; regulation in UK, 46–49, 65

embryo sexing, 40–41, 48–49, 206n6; accuracy of, 32–33, 89; as by-product of any PGD application, 36, 93, 156–57; PCR in, 35–36, 38, 48. *See also* fluorescence in situ hybridization (FISH); preimplantation genetic diagnosis (PGD); sperm sexing

embryo transfer, 48, 116, 134, 138–39; timing of, 36, 131–32, 135, 138, 145

emotionality, 102, 105, 125–26

Ericsson, Ronald, 61–62, 67

Ericsson method, 33, 206n7

ethical concerns: medical sex selection, 81, 86, 91, 93–94, 150–51, 159; MicroSort development, 86–88, 150; PGD development, 66–67, 85–88, 89, 93–94, 158–59; reproductive travel and, 116–17, 118. *See also* American Society for Reproductive Medicine (ASRM); biomedicalized sex selection, ethical debates; embryo production, ethical concerns

ethics, scholarship on, 193

European Society of Human Reproduction and Embryology (ESHRE): PGD Consortium, 49; Task Force on Ethics and Law, 93–94, 150

expectations, 106

extreme gender disappointment, 107–8

family balancer subject, 95, 96–101, 108–9, 110, 111, 114, 194

family balancing, 71; ASRM statements, 86–88; "complete" and "balanced" families as ideal, 13, 100–101, 151, 201, 203–4; data on, 165–66; defined, 4, 37, 97, 99; family planning and, 78, 96–97; female selection, 58, 99, 110, 154; gender

dreamer subject, 31, 95, 101–8, 109, 111, 114, 194; male selection, 126, 149, 150; reproductive travelers and, 126; term, 33, 37, 96, 97–100, 101–2; West/Rest binary and, 9, 70, 99, 186–87. *See also* biomedicalized sex selection; MicroSort

family balancing, as sex-neutral, 99, 110, 126, 151, 197, 203–4; UN statement, 149–50, 186–87. *See also* sex bias

family balancing indication, in MicroSort clinical trial: enrollment data, 5, 80; FDA prohibition of, 4, 34, 84, 94, 165; female selection, 154; GIVF IRB approval, 3–4, 34, 57–58, 80–82, 118; market-driven motivations, 4, 80; self-regulated enrollment policy, 81–82, 97–98, 99–102. *See also* MicroSort clinical trial

family formation narrative, 19–20

family identity, 11

family planner subject, 108, 111, 114

family planning, 77, 102, 125, 188, 202; contraception, synonymous with, 96, 100; family balancing and, 78, 96–97; individual sexual desire deemphasized, 100; sex-selective abortion and, 64–65. *See also* contraception; population control

family size, 76; "complete" and "balanced" families, as ideal, 13, 100–101, 151, 201, 203–4

farm animals. *See* agricultural industry

Fausto-Sterling, Anne, 10

FDA. *See* Food and Drug Administration (FDA)

female selection: abject anti-citizen and, 109–10; in agricultural industry, 41–42, 58–59; ASRM statements on, 87; to avoid genetic disease, 39–40, 48, 55; data on, 155; family balancing and, 58, 99, 110, 154; gender dreaming and, 103–4; in MicroSort clinical trial, 154; by Teigen and Legend, 12; X-sorts, 35, 208n1. *See also* family balancing, as sex-neutral; male selection; sex bias; sex ratios

feminism, 3, 74, 96, 110, 166; population control and, 7, 158, 173, 202–3

feminist intersectional perspective, 32, 197–98

feminist theory, perspective on NRTs, 20–30, 205n2; individual/social reproductive binary, 20–22; medicalization/population control reproductive binary, 20, 22–28; pro-/anti-natalist reproductive binary, 20, 28–30

fertility clinics, 31, 60, 76, 114; abortion clinics, 64, 172–73; ASRM statements, 85–89; complexity of opening as MicroSort lab, 141–42; infertility patients and sex selection patients in, 92; market-driven motivations in, 90–91, 95; private medical practice clinics, 65; self-regulation, 30, 78–79, 82, 197. *See also* Genetics & IVF Institute (GIVF); laboratories, off-shore, US-operated; reproductive travel, interclinic collaboration; reproductive travelers

Fertility Clinic Success Rate and Certification Act (1992), 154

"Fertility Ethics Authority Approves Sex Selection" (Kolata), 89, 158–59

Fertility Inc., term defined, 4. *See also* market-driven motivations; MicroSort; preimplantation genetic diagnosis (PGD)

Fertility Institutes' website, 136

fertility rates, 186

feticide, 174–79

FFWH (Forum for Women's Health), 6, 157–58

50:50 ratio of sperm sorts, 33, 62, 68

first baby sorts, 81, 99

Fishman, Jennifer, 193

Flavin, J., 174

flow cytometry, 42–44, 50; ASRM statements, 87, 94; bovine sperm sorting, 52, 54; DNA analysis and, 33, 34–35, 43; GIVF use, 55, 84; immobility and specialization of, 130; process, 34–35, 52, 130; sperm shape, 43, 44. *See also* sperm sexing

fluorescence in situ hybridization (FISH): micro-array CGH replaces, 36, 93, 132, 133, 156–57; PGD and, 35–36, 38, 49–50, 131, 133, 145, 156; process, 36, 131, 206n2; replaces PCR, 49–50; sperm sorting and, 50, 52, 63. *See also* preimplantation genetic diagnosis (PGD); sperm sexing

Food and Drug Administration (FDA): denies family balancing as indication in MicroSort trial, 4, 34, 84, 94, 165; Generations Ahead urges transparency about MicroSort, 164–66; GIVF withdraws premarket application, 129, 140, 154; MicroSort trial oversight, 34, 81, 82–84, 154, 205n4. *See also* Genetics & IVF Institute (GIVF), MicroSort trial and; MicroSort clinical trial

*Fortune* magazine, 5

Forum against Sex Determination and Sex Preselection (FASDSP), 6, 7, 157–58, 175

Forum for Women's Health (FFWH), 6, 157–58

Foucault, Michel, 18, 59, 73, 199

Fourth World Conference on Women (Beijing), 149

Franklin, Sarah, 46, 47, 60, 195

Franks, Trent, 162, 163

Fraser, Nancy, 172

#freepurvipatel campaign, 176

market narrative, 19–20. *See also* market-driven motivations

Hielingsdorf, Lizette, 109

Fugger, Edward, 45, 53, 97–98

Gammeltoft, Tine, 9

Gardner, Richard, 40

Garner, D. L., 41, 206n3

Garrard, Eve, 185, 188–89

gender-baby.com, 136–37

gender bias. *See* sex bias

*Gendercide: The Implications of Sex Selection* (Warren), 21

gender disappointment, 6, 102, 106–8

gender discrimination. *See* sex bias

gender dreamer subject, 31, 95, 101–8, 109, 111, 114, 194

gender dreaming: feminism and, 110; as fixation, 105–6

genderdreaming.com, 66–67, 104, 106–7, 110, 138

gendering fetuses as conferring personhood, 178

gender normativity, 10

genderselection.uk.com, 136

gender variety, 101. *See also* family balancing

gender vs. sex selection, 9–10

Generations Ahead (CGS spin off organization), 161–66; goal shifts, 165–66; Taking a Stand toolkit, 164, 166, 180; urges FDA's transparency about MicroSort, 164–66. *See also* "the campaign" (sex selection activism), history of

genetic disease prevention, Micro-Sort and: application limited to, 4, 33–34, 37–38, 39–40, 58, 59, 70; combined with PGD, 56, 59; FDA limits to, 4, 34, 84, 94, 165; first baby sorts, 99; FISH and, 50; USDA-GIVF research, 50, 51, 55, 80, 81. *See also* medical sex selection; MicroSort

genetic disease prevention, PGD and, 5, 33, 37–38, 39–40, 67, 70; accuracy of, 80; combined with MicroSort, 56, 59; crossover applications, 36, 93–94, 123, 150–51, 155–57; initial human use, 46; reproductive travelers and, 122–23; technology advances, 49; UK advocacy, 48–49. *See also* medical sex selection; PGD development, human use

Genetics and Public Policy Center, 155

Genetics & IVF Institute (GIVF), 45, 79–85; argues that prevented abortions constitutes public health need, 51, 84, 165–66; FDA premarket application withdrawn, 129, 140, 154; flow cytometry use, 55, 84; labs opened by, 34, 115, 128, 129, 131, 139–43; regulations, 83, 118; terminology used, 9, 98, 99, 101. *See also* in vitro fertilization (IVF); Schulman, Joseph D.; USDA-GIVF collaboration

Genetics & IVF Institute (GIVF), MicroSort trial and, 33, 80–83, 94, 205n4; approves family balancing as indication, 3–4, 34, 57–58, 80–82, 118; cedes authority to FDA, 82–83; self-regulated enrollment policy, 57, 81–82, 97–98, 99–102, 154; trial terminated, 139, 140. *See also* in vitro fertilization (IVF); MicroSort clinical trial

Ghai, Anita, 11

Gilbert, D., 37

Ginsburg, Faye, 193–94, 195

girl children. *See* female selection

Givan, Alice, 130

Gleicher, Norbert, 88–89

global bio-citizen subject. *See* biocitizenship

globalization, 74

*Global Politics of the IUD* (Takeshita), 59

India, stereotypes, 179, 190, 191, 202; "Replacing Myths" report, 187–88; by Western self-help authors, 69, 99, 109–10

India Abroad, 6, 158

Indian Americans, 113; Patel case, 174, 175–78. *See also* Asian Americans

Indian Express, 6, 158

individual desire, 9, 16–17, 74, 153, 201, 202–3; biopolitics and, 25–26, 27, 31, 96; biopower and, 59, 73, 199, 200; family balancing term, 100, 101; gender disappointment, 6, 102, 106–8; gender dreamer subject, 31, 95, 101–8, 109, 111, 114, 194; market-driven motivations, 75, 76, 77, 91; reproductive rights and privacy, 172, 173, 180; West/Rest binary, 150. *See also* neoliberalism

individual/social reproductive binary, 20–22, 28, 180, 198, 200

inequality terminology, 13–14

infanticide, 69, 108, 110

infertility, 18, 23, 41, 61, 137–38

infertility patients, 91–92, 156

ingender.com, 66–67, 98, 106, 129

inheritance motivation, 91, 112–13

Inhorn, Marcia C., 18, 123, 195

Inova Fairfax Hospital, 33–34, 55, 82

insemination: artificial, 41, 55, 57, 205n1; intrauterine (IUI), 60, 85, 88, 93, 127, 143

institutional review board (IRB), 33–34, 55, 81–82, 83, 89

interclinic collaboration. *See* reproductive travel, interclinic collaboration

International Conference on Population and Development (ICPD, Cairo, 1994), 3, 22, 65, 108, 184, 186–87; paradigm shift following, 24–25, 26; Programme of Action, 75, 148, 200

International Federation of Gynecology and Obstetrics (FIGO), 207n5

International Human Rights Clinic (University of Chicago), 168–69, 180

intracytoplasmic sperm injection (ICSI), 60–61, 146, 147

intrauterine devices (IUD), 59

intrauterine insemination (IUI), 60, 85, 88, 93, 127, 143

in vitro fertilization (IVF): batching cycles, 145; complexity, 58, 132, 145; cost, 88, 93, 104, 124; development of, 35, 40, 41, 42, 46–47, 85; embryo freezing, 132; first human birth, 41; invasiveness, 85, 88; normalization, 60; pig birth, 44; process, 35, 54, 58, 60–61, 132, 145; reproductive travel and, 132, 135, 145; staggered procedures, 36, 132, 138–39; success rate, 82, 93, 156, 195. *See also* embryo production through IVF; Genetics & IVF Institute (GIVF); preimplantation genetic diagnosis (PGD)

in vitro fertilization (IVF), PGD and, 58; data on, 5, 154–56; research and development, 41, 42, 46–47, 60, 85. *See also* preimplantation genetic diagnosis (PGD)

Jeffery, Patricia, 185

Jeffery, Roger, 185

Jesudason, Sujatha, 164

John, Mary, 191

Johnson, Lawrence, 40, 41, 43–45, 46, 55; FISH and, 50; pseudoscientific methods analysis by, 62; sort purity and, 53–54

Johnson, Martin H., 40

jurisdictional circumvention, 84. *See also* regulation and policy; reproductive travelers; reproductive travelers, legality issues

justice, 193, 196

Kalantry, Sital, 163, 183
Karabinus, David, 41, 44–45, 83, 101
Klass, Perri, 109
Knecht, Michi, 120
knowledge production and truth claims (data interpretation), 32, 171, 177, 202; abortion and, 9, 15, 153, 182–85; Almond and Edlund study, 162, 163, 164, 166, 169, 182; anti-abortion activism and, 15–16, 163, 166, 168–70; "Replacing Myths," 168–70, 180, 182, 186, 187–88; RJ response to sex selective abortion bans, 181–83, 187–90; sex ratios, 181–88, 191, 197. *See also* "the campaign" (sex selection activism), data and; data collection (raw data)
Kolata, Gina, 6, 89, 98–99, 158–59
Korea, 169, 187

laboratories, off-shore, US-operated, 4, 15, 31, 84; complexity of operating, 132–33, 141–42; GIVF opens, 34, 115, 128, 129, 131, 139–43; Guadalajara, 115–16, 119, 128–29, 131, 132, 145; initial opening, 140–43; inter-clinic collaboration, 119, 124–25, 127, 129–30, 131, 133–39, 197; lowered costs in, 124, 143; staffing, 130, 133, 141–42. *See also* fertility clinics; reproductive travel, interclinic collaboration; reproductive travelers
law. *See* regulation and policy
Lawrence Livermore National Laboratory, 42–43, 45
legal mosaicism, 118
Legend, John, 12
Leninist neoliberalism, 75

Li, Jiali, 29
liberated women subject, 108
lifestyle medicine and sex selection: defined, 11–12, 37. *See also* biomedicalized sex selection; family balancing; medical sex selection; PGD development, biomedicalized use
livestock. *See* agricultural industry
Look, Mary, 44
low-tech methods, 66–70, 104, 206n7. *See also* high-tech methods; pseudo-scientific methods
Luker, Kristin, 172, 173
Luna, Zaikiya, 172, 173

Malaysia, 141
male selection: data on, 155; family balancing and, 126, 149, 150; for inheritance reasons, 91, 112–13; injustice against women and, 21, 149; in non-West, 99, 109, 110; by reproductive travelers, 120; sex selective abortion, 64–65, 69; X-linked disease and, 40. *See also* female selection; sex bias; sex ratios; son preference
Mamo, Laura, 4, 14, 39, 193
Manavi Inc., 159, 160, 163
*Man-Made Women* (Corea et al.), 20
market-driven motivations, 14–15, 74–75, 102, 173, 197; behind family balancing indication, 4, 80; bio-citizens and, 95, 111–14; egg donation, 202; in fertility clinics, 90–91, 95; individual desire and, 75, 76, 77, 91; Micro-Sort development, 33, 79, 80–81, 92–95, 140, 143–44; PGD development, 80, 84–85, 90, 92–93; reproductive travelers and, 118–19; surrogacy, 202. *See also* neoliberalism
Max Planck Institute for Biochemistry, 41
Mbembe, Achille, 18

McCann, Carole, 177, 183–84

McGowan, Michelle L., 196

McLaren, A., 48–49

media coverage: on MicroSort births, 86, 98–99; on MicroSort clinical trial, 154; misrepresentational article on approval for PGD, 6, 89, 158–59

medicalization: abortion research and, 63–64, 65; of contraception, 65; gender disappointment and, 107–8; of pregnancy, 38, 68. *See also* biomedicalized sex selection

medicalization/population control reproductive binary, 20, 22–28

medical sex selection, 40, 43; campaign advocates limiting use to, 159, 161, 207n5; crossover applications, 36, 93–94, 123, 150–51, 155–57; defined, 11; ethics of, 81, 86, 91, 93–94, 150–51, 159; ICSI and, 61; as legitimate application, 5, 33, 46–49; MicroSort-PGD convergence, 37–39, 56–57, 59, 66–67, 194; pseudoscience, dissociated, 39, 61; sex selective abortion, dissociated, 39, 52, 64, 65, 194. *See also* biomedicalized sex selection; genetic disease prevention; MicroSort development, medicalized use; PGD development, biomedicalized use; PGD development, medicalized use

Medical Termination of Pregnancy Act (India), 175

Menon, Nivedita, 175

mental health issues, 107–8

Mexico, as reproductive travel hub, 31, 142; advantages of, 143–44; Guadalajara lab, 115–16, 119, 128–29, 131, 132, 145; process described, 145–48; profiles of travelers, 124. *See also* laboratories, off-shore, US-operated; reproductive travelers

micro-array CGH analysis (PGD), 36, 93, 132, 133, 156–57. *See also* fluorescence in situ hybridization (FISH)

MicroSort, 11; ASRM statements on, 86–88; as Beltsville Sperm Sexing Technology, 33, 40–45, 50–55, 62, 80, 206n3; cost, 143; data collection and publication, 5, 164–66; ESHRE statement on, 150; ethical concerns, 86–88, 150; family balancing introduced by, 37, 58; Generations Ahead urges transparency, 164–66; as high-tech, 38, 59–61, 66–71; immobility and specialization of technology, 127–31, 133–34; IUI and, 93, 143; media coverage on first births, 86, 98–99; medicalization redefinition, 30, 37–38, 40, 50, 58–59, 70, 194; naming, 55; patent, 84; process, 32–34, 50, 127–28; providers' comfort with, 91; vs. pseudoscientific methods, 61, 62–63, 194; regulatory inconsistency, 118. *See also* family balancing; genetic disease prevention, MicroSort and; Genetics & IVF Institute (GIVF); laboratories, off-shore, US-operated; MicroSort clinical trial; under MicroSort development; MicroSort-PGD convergence; preimplantation genetic diagnosis (PGD); sex selective abortion, MicroSort dissociated from; sperm sexing; USDA-GIVF collaboration

MicroSort clinical trial, 128; application limited to, 4, 33–34, 37–38, 39–40, 58, 59, 70; commercial development during, 33, 79, 80–81, 92–95, 140, 143–44; data collection in, 5, 80, 82, 94, 142, 154, 164–66; enrollment limit extended, 34, 83–84; FDA oversight, 34, 81, 82–84, 154, 205n4; flow cytometers and, 130; GIVF oversight (*See*

40; as legitimate, 5, 61–63, 66–67; MicroSort as adjunct, 37, 56–57, 59, 66–67; pseudo- and unscientific methods and, 61–63, 66–67; research pace, 40–41, 48; technical obstacles, 48

physicians. *See* providers

pigs, 41, 44, 45

Planned Parenthood, 172–73

*Planned Parenthood v. Casey* (1992), 162

Platoni, Kara, 96

Plowman, Dean, 80

PND. *See* prenatal diagnostic technologies (PND)

*Policing the National Body* (Silliman), 22

policy. *See* regulation and policy

polymerase chain reaction (PCR), 35–36, 38, 48–49

population control, 19–20, 73–77, 114; biopopulationism, 26–28, 32, 199–200; in China, 70, 74–77, 99, 109–10, 187–88; feminist activism and, 7, 158, 173, 202–3; infertility and, 18; medicalization binary, feminist perspective on, 20, 22–28; Orientalism and, 181, 183–84; RJ and, 7, 32, 173, 196–97; sex selective abortion, 24, 64–65, 66, 70, 75. *See also* contraception; family planning; India, population control in; sex ratios; sex selective abortion

Population Council, 64

population imbalance. *See* sex ratios

populationism, 27; biopopulationism, 26–28, 32, 199–200

population quality, 76

Population Research Institute, 162

population science, 181, 205n3

Potter, Daniel, 83

poverty, 173

Powell, Enoch, 48

power, 109, 111; biopower, 59, 73, 199, 200; stratified reproduction and, 193–94

Preconception and Prenatal Diagnostic Techniques Act (India, 1994), 65, 175

pregnancy: avoiding, 96; medicalization of, 38, 68; normalizing technological optimization, 60

preimplantation genetic diagnosis (PGD), 8, 11; anti-abortion activism and, 46–48, 65; ASRM Ethics Committee and, 6–7, 85–89, 158–59; cost, 93, 124, 156; crossover applications, 36, 93–94, 123, 150–51, 155–57; data collection and, 5, 154–57; defined, 35; DNA analysis and, 35–36, 49; family balancing term and, 98; FISH and, 35–36, 38, 49–50, 131, 133, 145, 156; as high-tech, 38, 59–61, 66–71; immobility and specialization of technology, 127, 131–34; media coverage, 6, 89, 99, 158–59; medicalization redefinition, 30, 37–38, 40, 46–50, 59, 70, 194; process, 32–33, 35–36, 42, 48–49, 131–32, 145–48; regulation of, 4, 35, 85, 87, 90, 94, 150; reproductive travel and, 6, 123, 124, 131–33, 139, 143; sex selection accuracy, 32, 57, 80, 89. *See also* biomedicalized sex selection; embryo; in vitro fertilization (IVF), PGD and; MicroSort; MicroSort-PGD convergence; under PGD development; sex selective abortion, PGD dissociated from

prenatal diagnostic technologies (PND), 46–49, 56–57; amniocentesis, 24, 47, 64–65, 69; GIVF and, 50; in India, 6, 64–65; PCR, 35–36, 38, 48–49; ultrasound, 24, 69. *See also* fluorescence in situ hybridization (FISH)

PRENDAs (Prenatal Nondiscrimination Acts), 178, 182

Preventing Gender-Biased Sex Selection (WHO statement), 149–50, 187 privacy rights, 153, 173, 203

pro-/anti-natalist reproductive binary, 16, 20, 28–30, 76–77

Proceedings of the National Academy of Sciences, 162

pro-choice activists, 173. *See also* anti-abortion activism

professional guidelines, 78, 85–89, 167, 207n5. *See also* American Society for Reproductive Medicine (ASRM)

PROGRESS, 41, 48

pro-life movement, 162. *See also* anti-abortion activism

protests. *See* "the campaign" (sex selection activism), history of

providers, 6; emotional labor of, 125–26; as entrepreneurs, 79; provider-client relationship, 75, 76; reproductive travel and, 112–13, 125–26, 139–40, 142–43, 144–48; self-regulation by, 90–95, 142–43, 207n5

pseudoscientific methods, 39, 61–63, 194; "low-tech" category and, 66–70, 104, 206n7. *See also* high-tech methods

Puri, Sunita, 161, 166, 169

rabbits, experiments with, 40, 44–45

Rabinow, Paul, 38

race, 113–14, 198–99; anti-abortion activism and, 7, 17, 32, 166, 173, 181, 191; campaign activism and, 169, 170–71, 179–80, 182, 197, 199; sex ratio and, 169–70; stratified reproduction and, 194; women of color, 18–19, 22, 173, 174. *See also* Asian Americans; Orientalism; reproductive justice (RJ); sex selective abortion bans, race and

radiation, effects on reproduction, 41–43

Rainsbury Clinic, 136

Rao, Mohan, 25

Rapp, Rayna, 193–94, 195

Raymond, Janice, 20, 21, 22–23

Reed, Catherine, 109

regulation and policy, 77, 207n5; campaign goals, 157–58, 161, 165, 167, 171, 180, 197; in China, 117, 198; decentering state authority, 15–16, 17, 118, 148, 151; FDA, 34, 81, 82–84, 154, 205n4; feticide law, 174–79; GIVF and, 82, 118; HFEA, 86, 118; in India, 65, 117, 174–75, 198; MicroSort clinical trial and, 83, 140; of PGD, 4, 35, 85, 87, 90, 94, 150; RJ activism, 172, 173, 199, 203; transnational inconsistency, 117, 118, 197; in UK, 46–49, 65, 117, 118, 122, 198. *See also* reproductive travelers; reproductive travelers, legality issues; self-regulation; sex selective abortion bans

regulation and policy, China, 117, 122, 198; population control, 70, 74–77, 109–11, 168, 181, 187–88

regulation and policy, India, 74, 75, 117, 122, 177, 198; population control, 161, 168, 202. *See also* India, population control in

regulatory absence, in US, 110, 117, 118, 154–55; clinics' interest in maintaining, 78–79, 82, 197; over PGD, 4, 35, 85, 87, 90, 94, 150. *See also* reproductive travelers

"Replacing Myths with Facts: Sex Selective Abortion Laws in the United States" (NAPAWF, ANSIRH, and International Human Rights Clinic report), 168–70, 180, 182, 186, 187–88

reproductive justice (RJ), 171–92; ACRJ, 164, 166, 172, 180; anti-abortion organizations and, 198–99; criminalization of reproduction and, 173–78; definition and aims, 22, 171–72, 173, 193, 196; developed

safety, ASRM statements on, 87–88
Saharso, Sawitri, 189–90
same-sex couples, 101
"savage baby killer" trope, 177, 178–79
Schulman, Joseph D., 45, 50, 57–58,
   79, 99, 118; family balancing term
   introduced by, 97. See also Genetics
   & IVF Institute (GIVF)
Schultz, Susanne, 25, 27
Schuppner, Nicole C., 90–91
Science, Technology, and Human Values
   (journal), 193
science and technology studies (STS)
   scholars, 28, 59, 193
Segal, Sheldon, 64–65
Seidel, G. E., Jr., 42, 206n3
self-help authors, 66–69, 93, 99, 102,
   104, 109–10. See also Thompson,
   Jennifer Merrill
self-regulation, 76, 117; campaign
   activism and, 167, 168; data absent
   or unpublished, 154–55; of fertility
   clinics, 30, 78–79, 82, 197; Micro-
   Sort trial enrollment policy, 57, 81–
   82, 97–98, 99–102, 154; professional
   associations guidelines, 85–89; by
   providers, 90–95, 142–43, 207n5.
   See also regulation and policy
Sen, Amartya, 184
sex bias, 3, 17, 100, 110, 126, 148–49;
   "Replacing Myths" and, 180; ste-
   reotype of Asian Americans, 155,
   163, 169, 183; West/Rest binary
   and, 11–12, 155, 194. See also family
   balancing, as sex-neutral; son
   preference
"Sexing Human Spermatozoa to
   Control Sex Ratios at Birth Is
   Now a Reality" (Edwards and
   Beard), 56
sex-linked disease. See genetic disease
   prevention; X-linked genetic disease prevention

sex ratios, 11, 98, 100, 117, 200; Asian
   Americans and, 162, 164, 169, 183;
   birth order and, 186; in China, 169,
   185, 187–88, 191; data, 164, 165,
   168, 169, 181–83; in India, 99, 169,
   184, 185, 187; knowledge production and, 181–88, 191, 197; race
   and, 169–70; sex selective abortions claimed to affect, 65, 149,
   166, 169, 184–85, 191
sex ratios in sperm samples. See
   sperm sexing
sex selection. See biomedicalized sex
   selection; medical sex selection
sex selection activism. See "the campaign" (sex selection activism),
   data and; "the campaign" (sex
   selection activism), history of
sex selection bans, 203. See also sex
   selective abortion bans
sex selection vs. gender selection,
   9–10
sex selective abortion, 11, 51, 63–70,
   157, 202; ASRM statements, 86, 94;
   awareness of, 24, 65; binaries in, 17,
   20–28; biomedicalized sex selection
   and, 24, 26, 30, 64, 150–51; claimed
   to affect sex ratios, 65, 149, 166,
   169, 184–85, 191; data on, 153, 165–
   66, 168–75; erased by high/low tech
   binary, 66, 69–70; feminist theory
   and, 20–21, 29–30; gender disappointment and, 107, 110; increase
   in, 74; in India, 64–65; male selection and, 64–65, 69; population
   control and, 24, 64–65, 66, 70, 75;
   son preference and, 6, 163, 182,
   187–88; West/Rest context, 14,
   69, 70, 97, 110, 188–90. See also
   abortion; abortion rights; population control
sex selective abortion, dissociation
   from, 5, 11, 86; biomedicalization

United States Constitution, 170
United States Department of Agriculture (USDA), 42, 43, 53, 62; Beltsville Sperm Sexing Technology (later MicroSort), 33, 40–45, 50–55, 62, 80, 206n3
United States Department of Energy, 41–43
United States Patent and Trademark Office (USPTO), 84
unknowable account, 153, 154. *See also* knowledge production and truth claims (data interpretation)
"Use of Reproductive Technology for Sex Selection for Nonmedical Reasons" (ASRM Ethics Committee), 94

valued reproduction, 16–17, 20, 202; devalued reproduction, 171, 177, 202
violence against women, 3, 6, 21, 158; feticide law and, 174–75
*Vogue* magazine, 109

Wadman, Meredith, 97–98
Wahlberg, Ayo, 9
Waldby, Catherine, 54
Warren, Mary Anne, 21
wealth, 111, 121–22
Weiss, Robin Elise, 66
Welch, Glenn, 52–53, 53–54, 62
welfare in India, 75
West/Rest binary, 13–15, 30; anti-abortion activism and, 188, 191; family balancing and, 9, 99, 186–87; individual desire and, 150; male selection and, 99, 109, 110; nonmedical sex selection and,

116–17, 149–50; Orientalism, 13–14, 32, 194; sex bias and, 11–12, 155, 194; sex selective abortion and, 14, 69, 70, 97, 110, 188–90
white women, 18–19
Whittaker, A. M., 123–24
Wilkinson, Stephen, 185, 188–89
Wilson, Kalpana, 177
Winckler, Edwin A., 75
Winston, Robert, 48
Wise, David, 83
women, 74; male selection as injustice against, 21, 149; violence against, 3, 6, 21, 158, 174–75
women of color, 18–19; abortion rights and, 173; criminalization of pregnant, 174; scholarship by, on individual/social reproductive binary, 22
World Conference on Women (Beijing, 1995), 3
World Health Organization (WHO), 149–50

X-linked genetic disease prevention: females selected, 39–40, 49; MicroSort indications, 34, 56, 57–58; PGD development, 37, 46, 56–58; USDA/GIVF research, 51, 55, 57–58, 80–81. *See also* genetic disease prevention; human medicine
X-sorts, 35, 208n1

Yeung, Miriam, 182, 183, 184, 187
Y-sorts, 48–49

"0+12" method, 67
Zola, Irving, 22

**Feminist Technosciences**

Rebecca Herzig and Banu Subramaniam, *Series Editors*

*Figuring the Population Bomb: Gender and Demography in the Mid-Twentieth Century*, by Carole R. McCann

*Risky Bodies & Techno-Intimacy: Reflections on Sexuality, Media, Science, Finance*, by Geeta Patel

*Reinventing Hoodia: Peoples, Plants, and Patents in South Africa*, by Laura A. Foster

*Queer Feminist Science Studies: A Reader*, edited by Cyd Cipolla, Kristina Gupta, David A. Rubin, and Angela Willey

*Gender before Birth: Sex Selection in a Transnational Context*, by Rajani Bhatia